The Authorities

Powerful Wisdom from Leaders in the Field

LYNNE NIEPAGE

Just4Mie Pole Therapy

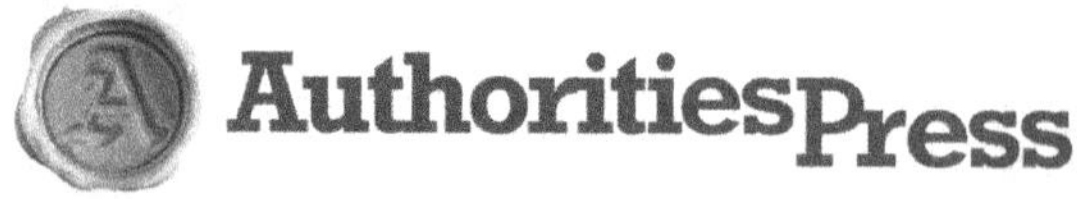

Copyright © 2017 Authorities Press

ISBN-13:978-1978273962
ISBN-10:1978273967

Limits of Liability and Disclaimer of Warranty

The author and publisher shall not be liable for your misuse of the enclosed material. This book is strictly for informational and educational purposes.

Warning – Disclaimer

The purpose of this book is to educate and entertain. The author and/or publisher do not guarantee that anyone following these techniques, suggestions, tips, ideas, or strategies will become successful. The author and/or publisher shall have neither liability nor responsibility to anyone with respect to any loss or damage caused, or alleged to be caused, directly or indirectly by the information contained in this book.

Medical Disclaimer
The medical or health information in this book is provided as an information resource only, and is not to be used or relied on for any diagnostic or treatment purposes. This information is not intended to be patient education, does not create any patient-physician relationship, and should not be used as a substitute for professional diagnosis and treatment.

Publisher
Authorities Press
Markham, ON
Canada

Printed in Canada and the United States.

FOREWORD

Experts are to be admired for their knowledge, but they often remain unrecognized by the general public because they save their information and insights for paying customers and clients. There are many experts in a given field, but their impact is limited to the handful of people with whom they work.

Unlike experts, authorities share their knowledge and expertise far more broadly, so they make a big impact on the world. Authorities become known and admired as leading experts and, as such, typically do very well economically and professionally. Most authorities are also mature enough to know that part of the joy of monetary success is the accompanying moral and spiritual obligation to give back.

Many people want to learn and work with well-respected and generous authorities, but don't always know where to find them. They may be known to their peers, or within a specific community, but have not had the opportunity to reach a wider audience. At one time, they might have submitted a proposal to the For Dummies or Chicken Soup for the Soul series of books, but it's now almost impossible to get accepted as a new author in such branded book series.

It is more than fitting that Raymond Aaron, an internationally known and respected authority in his own right, would be the one to recognize the need for a new venue in which authorities could share their considerable knowledge with readers everywhere. As the only author ever to be included in both of the book series mentioned above, Raymond has had the opportunity to give back and he understands how crucial it is for authorities to have a platform from which to share their expertise.

I have known and worked with Raymond for a number of years and consider him a valued friend and talented coach. He knows how to spot talented and knowledgeable people and he desires to see them prosper. Over the years, success coaching and speaking engagements around the world have made it possible for Raymond to meet many of these talented authorities. He recognizes and relates to their passion and enthusiasm for what they do, as well as their desire to share what they know. He tells me that's why he created this new nonfiction branded book series, The Authorities.

Dr. Nido Qubein
President, High Point University

TABLE OF CONTENTS

IV

INTRODUCTION

This book introduces you to *The Authorities* — individuals who have distinguished themselves in life and in business. Authorities make a big impact on the world. Authorities are leaders in their chosen fields. Authorities typically do very well financially, and are evolved enough to know that part of the joy of monetary success is the accompanying social, moral and spiritual obligation to give back.

Authorities are not just outstanding. They are also *known* to be outstanding.

This additional element begins to explain the difference between two strategic business and life concepts — one that seems great, but isn't, and the other that fills in the essential missing gap of the first.

The first concept is "the expert."

What is an expert? The real definition is …

EXPERT: *a person who knows stuff*

People who have attained a very senior academic degree (like a PhD or an MD) definitely know stuff. People who read voraciously and retain what they read definitely know stuff. Unfortunately, just because you know stuff does not mean that anyone respects the fact that you do. Even though some experts are successful, alas, most are not — because knowing stuff is not enough.

Well, then, what is the missing piece?

What the expert lacks, "the authority" has. The authority both knows stuff and is *known* to know stuff. So, more simply …

AUTHORITY: *a person who is known as an expert*

The difference is not subtle. The difference is not merely semantic. The difference is enormous.

When it comes to this subject, there are actually three categories in which people fall:

- People who don't know much and are unsuccessful in life and in business. Most people fall in this category.

- People who know stuff, but still don't leave much of a footprint in the world. There are a lot of people like this.

- Experts who are also *known* as experts become authorities and authorities are always wondrously successful. Authorities are able to contribute more to humanity through both their chosen work and their giving back.

This book is about the highest category, *The Authorities* — people who have reached the peak in their field and are known as such.

If you are interested in gaining confidence while having fun, you must read Lynne Niepage's chapter. With her expert guidance and engaging personality, Lynne will make you feel right at home as you learn about her Yoga and Pole™ studio. At Yoga and Pole™, you will be welcomed into a comfortable, inviting atmosphere where you will discover your inner goddess! Join Lynne as she shares exactly what an 'everyday woman' can become with a little 'pole therapy': confident, sexy, and incredibly fit! Read each chapter carefully to learn and to see the business potential that may be possible between yourself and each one of *The Authorities*. You may well be able to become their client or, possibly, do business with them in other ways.

They are *The Authorities*. Learn from them. Connect with them. Let them uplift you. Learning from them and working with them is the secret ingredient for success which may well allow you to rise to the level of Authority soon.

To be considered for inclusion in a subsequent edition of *The Authorities*, register to attend a future event at www.aaron.com/events where you will be interviewed and considered.

Find Your True Self with Yoga and Pole

LYNNE NIEPAGE

A few years ago, I visited Las Vegas for a NASCAR event. One evening my friend's brother drove a group of us in his car to meet their aunt for dinner. I twisted around in the front seat so I could better see my friends in the back seat and chatted excitedly when we were stopped at a stoplight. We were at the stoplight on Flamingo Road heading away from the Las Vegas Strip when an underage, impaired driver hit us doing between 60-70 mph.

The impact on the rear driver's side pushed us forward about one and a half car lengths. It sounded like a bomb had gone off and debris flew everywhere as the driver bounced off a Mustang convertible beside us and went airborne over us. Yes, I saw the whole underside of his car as it went over us. There was axle grease up the side of our car!

The impaired driver was taken away by ambulance; he survived the accident and we heard he eventually ended up skipping the country to avoid prosecution. Some witnesses stopped after the accident and waited with us until the investigator arrived. They said the driver who hit us was passed out in his car at a previous stoplight. I do not know if someone honked at him causing him to slam his foot on the accelerator before passing out again or just what happened. The investigator said the driver never even put on the brakes before hitting us!

The post-accident debris field was probably 100 square feet or more, leaving five lanes closed for about three hours. First the firemen arrived, then the paramedics, then the police, followed by the investigator. Finally, the flatbeds came to remove our car and the drunk's car (the Mustang was still drivable).

I was happy and rather amazed that I was alive and basically intact, but I never did make it to NASCAR. Shock is a funny thing. I recall saying to the girl in the Mustang, "Aren't you glad the Mustang convertible was the first convertible ever to receive the 5 Star crash safety rating?"

Unfortunately, since I was twisted in my seat when the accident occurred, I ended up with a protruded lumbar disc, a concussion, a dent in my skull, and whiplash. The following months were filled with brain and back doctors, a chiropractor, imaging, and epidural injections. But me being the typical female, I was worried about the ever-increasing size of my butt. You see, I have less than stellar eating habits (I like tasty food), and in the past, I had used running to burn calories so I could eat the foods I like. With the damage to my spine, running was not only painful but not advised. Of course, it was a vicious circle because the more weight I gained from lack of exercise, the more my back hurt which made exercise more painful.

I decided to find something new and low-impact that would keep me interested so that I would stick with it long enough to make a positive difference in my body. I decided to try pole dancing. I mean, doesn't everyone? It piqued my interest and it looked fun, so I decided to give it a try. I went online to find a local studio and signed up for a class.

My trial class was the following Saturday. I awoke that morning excited and a little anxious. Would my back be able to handle pole dancing? Would I look stupid doing it? Would everyone else be better than me? Would I even like it?

Would I stick with it?

I squared my shoulders, gave myself a pep talk, and headed out. The class began with introductions and, happily for me, with gentle stretches and moves to warm up the spine and body. When the instructor ended the class, I was surprised it was over. Time had flown by and I felt great! I was surprised that I not only felt better physically, but I felt better emotionally too. I was hooked!

After that first class, I convinced my friend, who had been in the car accident with me, to sign up for the next session. It was enlightening to discover that we both enjoyed the class even though our body types are very different. Some things came easier to me and some were easier for her, but we both saw improvements in ourselves. I have since learned that this is an experience that opens your eyes to each individual's unique beauty. Every person in the class is on their own journey, each different, but we all share a supportive experience.

The more I attended classes over the following months, the better and stronger I felt. As I progressed, my core strengthened and I became more flexible which, as it turns out, was incredibly good for my back. I always left the studio feeling better than when I arrived. I now refer to it as Pole Therapy!

JUST4MIE

I received a job transfer back home with my day job and decided to open my own studio. That is how Just4MiE was born! Contrary to the beliefs of some, this kind of pole dancing empowers women. When you take a pole dancing class, your mind and body stretch and develop. You will learn to respect your body's strengths and appreciate your own unique beauty as you gain confidence and self-worth. I created Just4MiE for every woman, no matter her age, shape, size, or fitness level. My desire is that every woman experience the joy and satisfaction I felt after my first class.

After several years and a flood (yes, flood, but that is another story), I decided that I did not want to pay an unresponsive landlord the high ticket rent anymore. So, I developed a plan. My lease was up for renewal the following spring and they required six months' notice if I planned to cancel. It was summer, so that only gave me a few months to put my plan in motion.

I was going to sell my house and buy a live/work building where I could have the studio in the commercial space and live above it. I would be close to the studio; my entire commute would be down a set of stairs. It was brilliant! The only obstacle left was to find one.

It turns out that finding a live/work unit in the right location with suitable ceiling height and layout (both studio and home) was harder than I expected. I finally found a new build that would work. It was perfect and the close date matched up with the last month at the current studio!

Unfortunately, I was twentieth in line and they were sold before my turn came up. Not to be deterred, I awaited the next release and made sure I did not miss out this time by sleeping in the parking lot the night before the release! Even showing up at noon the day before the release I was twenty-sixth in line and there were only ten units available. Of those ten, only four were suitable for a studio and only two had the layout I wanted.

The drill was to check in every four hours to keep your place in line, but I and many others were not going to take the chance of missing roll call, so we set up camp in the parking lot! Roll call after roll call the numbers dwindled. At the nine o'clock AM opening I was in sixth position. I got my unit of choice!

The close date meant I would be closed for three months, which was not ideal, but I was happy to have what would become the new studio. The last newly-built home I purchased had no construction delays, so I was not prepared for what ended up being a sixteen-month delay!

When the first delay occurred, I reached out to a fellow studio owner to see if she minded that I take classes at her studio so I could keep dancing. Turns out, she did mind. Then my sister suggested yoga and I agreed it was a perfect idea. So, I used the construction delays to get my yoga teaching certification.

Yoga is the perfect complement to pole dancing! Both get you to pay attention to your movement, physical and mental balance, mindfulness, breathing, strength, and flexibility. Adding aerial yoga, as well, gives you a natural progression from the earth to the air!

At Just4MiE I decided to offer yoga classes along with pole dance classes; therefore, the operating name had to change. Yoga and Pole™ was born! The health benefits of yoga are well-known and extensive. Yoga not only increases flexibility and builds muscle, but it also can do the following when practiced regularly: lower blood pressure, improve bone health, increase blood flow, improve sleep, balance, and focus, among many additional benefits.

Pole dance and yoga complement each other well. In pole dancing you will use muscles you may not have known you had! I have yoga classes that are designed specifically to stretch and strengthen muscles used in my pole dance classes. I also incorporate yoga in my pole dance classes via the warm-up, breathing technique while holding poses, and the cool down. The combination of grounding meditation and yoga, the sassy fun of sensual dance, and the strength-building of moves on the pole ensure a uniquely fun way to be active and build confidence. It is the workout that does not feel like work!

If you are unfamiliar with the concept of pole fitness, you may be a bit shocked by the idea. Pole-dancing often gets a bad rap but it is time to stop associating pole dance with stripping. Pole dance is a complete workout that combines cardiovascular fitness with resistance training and flexibility. You will be impressed as you witness changes in your strength, grace, and, yes, sensuality. You can soon be in the best shape of your life!

Many people think the only reason to learn pole-dancing is to perform for others. So wrong! The women who attend my classes do so for themselves. It is empowering and improves your self-image, which is a positive thing. If you happen to share what you have learned, it is a gift not a requirement!

Just4MiE's studio is designed for the comfort of my clients. In the beginning, some women are uncomfortable with themselves and worry about seeing their jiggly bits in the mirror, so I offer to cover the mirrors. I want women to focus on how they feel on the inside, not how they look on the outside. My clients learn to focus on their form by listening to my voice and feeling the movement in their body rather than focusing on what they see in the mirror.

Soon they begin seeing themselves differently as their body image changes. They no longer notice their jiggly bits; they notice a strong, confident woman who is willing to work hard to feel better inside and out.   While working on the outside, I also encourage women to work on the inside by challenging their limiting beliefs about themselves.

A limiting belief is any idea or belief you hold to be true that holds you back in some way.   We all have them, but some of us never acknowledge them. Once acknowledged, a limiting belief can be challenged and eradicated. This may sound simple, but it is not as easy as it sounds.

Pay attention to what you say to yourself through the day.   Is it something you would say to the person sitting next to you? If not, do not say it to yourself. Is it mostly positive or mostly negative? For every negative thought, substitute a positive one. The longest relationship you will ever have in your life is with yourself. Make it a great relationship! Be kind to yourself.

When I think of limiting beliefs, Beverly comes to mind. She was practically dragged to a trial class by a friend.   Beverly was not an ideal weight when I first met her but, more importantly, she did not believe she deserved to feel good about herself. At the beginning of a trial class there are often nervous giggles, but Beverly did not crack a smile. By the end of class, she had relaxed and seemed to be enjoying herself. I was thrilled when she signed up and continued to attend regularly.

By practicing meditation along with physical fitness Beverly became aware of the limiting beliefs she had about herself and began to challenge them. She tuned in to her inner dialogue and realized just how hostile she was to herself. She began to change her inner dialogue by giving herself grace and learning to be kind to herself.

Beverly has since lost weight and toned up; now she likes how she looks on the outside. However, she loves the confident woman she has become on the inside! The limiting belief that she is not deserving still pops in from time to time, but she is now aware of these negative thoughts and does not allow them to remain for long.

MARCIE

Marcie is one of the most beautiful people you can imagine. Her angelic looks and amazingly fit body make you think she must have some tragic flaw in her personality to balance it all out. But you would be wrong; she also has a very sweet, selfless nature and goes out of her way to help others.

One summer evening, Marcie first came to the studio for a bachelorette party. Afterward, she asked me about the timing of the first session of the next year since she had commitments that would prevent her from attending the fall sessions. Typically, when someone puts off starting a session, I don't expect to see them again but that did not happen with Marcie. Come the new year, she was there and thereafter attended weekly for years!

As I got to know her, I realized Marcie did not see herself as I, or others, saw her. Through months of classes, I saw her become more comfortable with her body and her femininity. I still remember the joyous expression on her face when she completed one of her special assignment graduation dances; she had finally gotten outside of her head and danced her emotions!

This was also an important reminder for me that what is going on outside of a person is not always a reflection of what is happening on the inside. Each person's journey is different and relative to their own true self, not to yours.

Dancing to what you feel and relating to the music instead of thinking about what you look like or what others will think is truly liberating! It can allow you to release painful or negative emotions and, conversely, it can amplify happy, joyous emotions. We have methods for helping you achieve this liberation, but I will not divulge those secrets here. (The "liberating" is referring to your mind and emotions, not body parts, as there is never any nudity in the studio!)

It is natural when you are in a supportive environment like our studio to feel comfortable sharing deeper emotions and life experiences than you ever would at the local gym! The studio is like Vegas; what happens in the studio, stays in the studio!

IT IS A PROCESS

Another student, Jan, taught me a valuable lesson. When a competition organizer came to the studio and asked if I had any students that would be competing in the upcoming pole dance weekend, I responded that I would post the flyer, but I doubted that any students would compete.

I was projecting my limiting belief onto my students. I did not like to be the center of attention and assumed that my students would not be interested in competing until they had mastered the sport. When I mentioned the competition to some students, Jan did show a hint of interest. Luckily, I realized my mistake and fully supported her preparation for the competition.

I am so grateful that I did not let my fears get in the way of supporting Jan and her entry into the competition. Yes, she did get a medal in her category but that is not the point. Her dance was so beautiful and very moving; it reminded me how important the emotional component is in dance and that you should not hold back just because you are "in process." I thank Jan for reminding me of that!

We have a tough time being "in process." We want to make changes and have the results yesterday! We have difficulty settling for anything less than perfection, which starts the cycle of self-doubt when we are human and do not master change on the first (or second, or tenth) try. We are usually our own worst critics too. We often feel that we must master a move, skill, or task before we can be happy with ourselves. This is not true! Be content to be in process; do not wait for the final accomplishment to feel your joy. Be proud of each step you take towards your goal!

I am sure you have seen one of those picture progressions showing what the model really looked like followed by the filtered lenses and Photoshop steps needed to get the final advertisement. Or I know you have seen a twenty-year-old model demonstrating the benefits of an anti-wrinkle cream in the pages of a magazine. How about the pudgy, pale, sad guy who develops muscles and a tan in 'just four weeks' by trying the latest diet and exercise fad? It is no surprise that we are rarely successful when we try to get the advertised results immediately upon using the product or service. It should come as no surprise that you may feel inadequate when you see your image in a mirror; you are comparing yourself to something that does not even exist in nature!

I think that there should be truth in advertising to the degree that only people who use the product or service advertise it. Do not get me wrong, I am all about aspiring to be the best you can be. I just think the image of what that is should be realistic!

There is no "one size fits all" self-improvement plan because we are all unique. We each have unique body shapes and contours, facial features, life experiences, and genetics; we all have our own unique beauty. Let your unique beauty shine!

Nothing is more attractive than a woman who is confident and comfortable with who she is. I lost my confidence after my car accident. Not being able to run took a mental toll just as it took a physical one. I missed those endorphins! I missed feeling good after a hard workout!

Words cannot express how much my life has improved since I tried that first pole dance class. Learning to do something physically challenging that I never dreamed I could do was incredibly empowering. Obviously, I am passionate about pole fitness and yoga because I opened my own studio and now share my love with others. If you would like to find a Yoga and Pole™ in your neighborhood, check my website Yoga and Pole™ for a location where you will always get the special intimacy you feel at the friendly neighborhood studio and where you will find your true self! If you are considering opening your own studio, contact me for Yoga and Pole™ franchise information.

During a Yoga and Pole™ by Just4MiE class you will you will meet and make new friends while participating in a meditation and a workout which can include yoga, dance, and/or pole! I would love for you to join me! If you cannot get to Yoga and Pole™ in your neighborhood, my advice is to try a few different studios and instructors in your area to find the best fit for you. Visit my website, www.yogaandpole.com, then sign up for my newsletter at http://bit.ly/2ueMUoT.

Branding Small Business

RAYMOND AARON

Branding is an incredibly important tool for creating and building your business. Large companies have been benefiting from branding ever since people first started selling things to other people. Branding made those businesses big.

If you're a small business owner, you probably imagine that small companies are different and don't need branding as much as large companies do. Not true. The truth is small businesses need branding just as much, if not more, than large companies.

Perhaps you've thought about branding, but assumed you'd need millions of dollars to do it properly, or that branding is just the same thing as marketing. Nothing could be further from the truth.

Marketing is the engine of your company's success. Branding is the fuel in that engine.

In the old days, salespeople were a big part of the selling process. They recommended one product over another and laid out the reasons why it was better. Salespeople had credibility because they knew about all the products, and customers often took the advice they had to offer.

Today, consumers control the buying process. They shop in big box stores, super-sized supermarkets, and over the Internet — where there are no salespeople. Buyers now get online and gather information beforehand. They learn about all the products available and look to see if there really is any difference between them. Consumers also read reviews and check social media to see if both the company and the product are reputable. In other words, they want to know what the brand is all about.

The way of commerce used to be: "Nothing happens till something is sold." Today it's: "Nothing happens till something is branded!"

DEFINING A BRAND

A brand is a proper name that stands for something. It lives in the consumer's mind, has positive or negative characteristics, and invokes a feeling or an image. In short, it's a person's perception of a product or a company.

When all goes well, consumers associate the same characteristics with a brand that the company talks about in its advertising, public relations, marketing and sales materials. Of course, when a product doesn't live up to what the company says about it, the brand gets a bad reputation. On the other hand, if a product or service over-delivers on the promises made, the brand can become a superstar.

RECOGNIZING BRANDING AND ITS CHARACTERISTICS

Branding is the science and art of making something that isn't unique, unique. Branding in the marketplace is the same as branding on a ranch. On a ranch, ranchers use branding to differentiate their cattle from every other rancher's cattle (because all cattle look pretty much the same). In the marketplace, branding is what makes a product stand out in a crowd of similar products. The right branding gets you noticed, remembered and sold — or perhaps I should say bought, because today it is all about buying, not selling.

There are four main characteristics of branding that make it an integral part of the marketing and purchasing process.

1. Branding makes you trustworthy and known

Branding makes a product more special than other products. With branding, a normal, everyday product has a personality, and a first and last name, and people know who you are.

In today's marketplace, most products are, more or less, just like their competition. Toilet paper is toilet paper, milk is milk, and a grocery store by any other name is still a grocery store. However, branding takes a product and makes it unique. For example, high-quality drinking water is available from just about every tap in the Western world and it's free, but people pay good money for it when it comes in a bottle. Branding takes bottled water and makes Evian.

Furthermore, every aspect of your brand gives potential customers a feeling or comfort level that they associate with you. The more powerful and positive that feeling is, the more easily and more frequently they will want to do business with you and, indeed, will do business with you.

2. Branding differentiates you from others

Strong branding makes you better than your competition, and makes your product name memorable and easy to remember. Even if your product is absolutely the same as every other product like it, branding makes it special. Branding makes it the first product a consumer thinks about when deciding to make a purchase.

Branding also makes a product seem popular. Everyone knows about it, which implicitly says people like it. And, if people like it, it must be good.

3. Branding makes you worth more money

The stronger your branding is, the more likely people are willing to spend that little bit extra because they believe you, your product, your service, or your business are worth it. They may say they won't, but they will. They do it all the time.

For example, a one-pound box of Godiva chocolates costs about $40; the same weight of Hershey's Kisses costs about $4. The quality of the chocolate isn't ten times greater. The reason people buy Godiva is that the brand Godiva means "gift" whereas the brand Hershey means "snack". Gifts obviously cost more than snacks.

4. Branding pre-sells your product

In the buying age, people most often make the decision on which products to pick up before they walk into the store. The stronger the branding, the more likely people are to think in terms of your product rather than the product category. For example, people are as likely, maybe even more likely, to add Hellmann's to the shopping list as they are to write down simply mayo. The same is true for soda, ketchup, and many other products with successful, strong branding.

Plus, as soon as a shopper gets to the shelf, branding can provide a quick reminder of what products to grab in a few ways:

- An icon or logo
- A specific color
- An audio icon

BRANDING IN A SMALL BUSINESS

Big companies spend millions of dollars on advertising, marketing, and public relations (PR) to build recognition of a new product name. They get their selling messages out to the public using television, radio, magazines, and the Internet. They can even throw money at damage control when necessary. The strategies for branding are the same in a small business, but the scale, costs, and a few of the tactics change.

Make your brand name work harder

The name of a small business can mean everything in terms of branding. Your brand name needs to work harder for your business than you do. It's the first thing a prospective customer sees, and it is how they will remember you. A brand name has to be memorable when spoken, and focused in its meaning. If the name doesn't represent what consumers believe about a product and the company that makes it, then that brand will fail.

In building your product's reputation and image, less is often significantly more. Make sure the name you choose immediately gives a sense of what you do.

Large corporations have millions of dollars to take a meaningless brand name and make it stand for something. Small businesses don't, so use words that really mean something. Strive for something interesting and be right on point. You don't need to be boring.

Plumbers, for example, would do well setting themselves apart with names like "The On-Time Plumber" or "24/7 Plumbing". The same is true for electricians, IT providers, or even marketing consultants. Plenty of other types of business are so general in nature they just don't work hard enough in a business or product name.

Even the playing field: The Net

The Internet has leveled the playing field for small businesses like nothing else. You can use the Internet in several ways to market your brand:

Website: Developing and maintaining a website is easier than ever. Anyone can find your business regardless of its size.

Social Media: Facebook and Twitter can promote your brand in a cost-effective manner.

BUILDING YOUR BRAND WITH THE BRANDING LADDER

Even if you do everything perfectly the first time (and I don't know anyone who does), branding takes time. How much time isn't just up to you, but you can speed things along by understanding the different levels of branding, as well as the business and marketing strategies that can get you to the top.

Introducing the Branding Ladder

Moving through the levels of branding is like climbing a ladder to the top of the marketplace. The Branding Ladder has five distinct rungs and, unlike stairs, you can't take them two at a time. You have to take them in order, and some businesses spend more time on each rung than others.

You can also think of the Branding Ladder in terms of a scale from zero to ten. Everyone starts at zero. If you properly climb the ladder, you can end up at 12 out of 10. The Branding Ladder below shows a special rung at the top of the ladder that can take your business over the top. The following section explains the Branding Ladder and how your small business can move up it.

THE BRANDING LADDER	
Brand Advocacy	**12/10**
Brand Insistence	**10/10**
Brand Preference	**3/10**
Brand Awareness	**1/10**
Brand Absence	**0/10**

Rung 1: Living in the void

Your business, in fact every business, starts at the bottom rung, which is called brand absence, meaning you have no brand whatsoever except your own name. On a scale of one to ten, brand absence is, of course, zero. That's the worst place to live and obviously the most difficult entrepreneurially. The good news is that the only way is up.

Ninety-seven percent of businesses live on this rung of the Branding Ladder. They earn far less than they want to earn, far less than they should earn, and far less than they would earn if they did exactly the same work under a real brand.

Rung 2: Achieving awareness

Brand awareness is a good first step up the ladder to the second rung. Actually, it's really good, especially because 97 percent of businesses never get there. You want people to be aware of you. When person A speaks to person B and says, "Have you heard of "The 24/7 Plumber?" You want the answer to be "yes".

On that scale of one to ten, however, brand awareness is only a one. It's better than nothing, but not that much better. Although people know of your brand, being aware doesn't mean that they are interested in buying it. Coca Cola drinkers know about Pepsi, but they don't drink it.

Rung 3: Becoming the preferred brand

Getting to the third rung, brand preference, is definitely a real step up. This rung means that people prefer to use your product or service rather than that of your competition. They believe there is a real difference between you and others, and you're their first choice. This rung is a crucial branding stage for parity products, such as bottled water and breakfast cereals, not to mention plumbers, electricians, lawyers, and all the others. Brand preference is clearly better than brand awareness, but it's less than halfway up the ladder.

Car rental companies represent a perfect example of why brand preference may not be enough. When someone lands at an airport and needs to rent a car on the spot, he or she may go straight to the preferred rental counter. If that company has a car available, it's a sale. However, if all the cars for that company have been rented, the person will move to the next rental kiosk without much thought, because one rental car is just as good as another.

Exerting Brand Preference needs to be easy and convenient

If all you have is brand preference, your business is on shaky ground and you can lose business for the feeblest of reasons. Very few people go to a second or third supermarket just to find their favorite brand of bottled water. Similarly, a shopper may prefer one store over another but, if both stores sell the same products, he or she will often go to the closest store even if it is not the better liked one. The reason for staying nearby does not need to be a dramatic one — the shopper may simply be tired, on a tight schedule, or not in the mood to travel.

Rung 4: Making it you and only you

When your customers are so committed to your product or service that they won't accept a substitute, you have reached the fourth rung of the Branding Ladder. All companies strive to reach this place, called brand insistence.

Brand insistence means that someone's experience with a product in terms of performance, durability, customer service, and image has been sufficiently exceptional. As a result, the product has earned an incredible level of loyalty.

If the product isn't available where the customer is, he or she will literally not buy something else. Rather, the person will look for the preferred product elsewhere. Can you imagine what a fabulous place this is for a company to be? Brand insistence is the best of the best, the perfect ten out of ten, the whole ball of wax.

Apple is a perfect example of brand insistence

Apple users don't just think, they know in their heads and hearts, that anything made by Apple is technologically-advanced, user-friendly, and just all-around superior. Committed to everything Apple, Mac users won't even entertain the thought that a PC may have positive attributes.

Apple people love everything about their Macs, iPads, iPhones, the Mac stores and all those apps. When the company introduces a new product, many of its brand-insistent fans actually wait in line overnight to be one of the first to have it. Steve Jobs is one of their idols.

Considering one big potential problem

Unfortunately, you can lose brand insistence much more quickly than you can achieve it. Brand-insistent customers have such high expectations that they can be disillusioned or disappointed by just one bad product experience. You also have to consistently reinforce the positives because insistence can fade over time. Even someone who has bought and re-bought a specific brand of car for the last 20 years can decide it's just time for a change. That's how fickle the world is.

At ten out of ten, brand insistence may seem like the top rung of the ladder, but it's not. One rung is actually better, and it involves getting your brand-insistent customers to keep polishing your brand for you.

Rung 5: Getting customers to do the work for you

Brand advocacy is the highest rung on the ladder. It's better than ten out of ten because you have customers who are so happy with your product that they want everyone to know about it and use it. Think of them as uber-fans. Not only do they recommend you to friends and family, they also practically shout your praises from the rooftops, interrupt conversations among strangers to give their opinion, and tell everyone they meet how fantastic you are. Most companies can only aspire to this level of customer satisfaction. Apple is one of the few large corporations in recent history that has brand advocates all over the world.

- Brand advocacy does the following five extraordinary things for your company. Brand advocacy:

- Provides a level of visibility that you couldn't pay for if you tried. Brand advocates are so enthusiastic they talk about you all the time, and reach people in ways general media and public relations can't. You get great visibility because they make sure people actually listen.

- Delivers free advertising and public relations. Companies love the extra super-positive messaging, all for free.

- Affords a level of credibility that literally can't be bought. Brand advocates are more than just walking testimonials. They are living proof that you are the best.

- Provides pre-sold prospective customers. Advocate recommendations carry so much weight that they are worth much more than plain referrals. They deliver customers ready and committed to purchasing your product or service.

- Increases profits exponentially. Brand advocates are money-making machines for your business because they increase sales and decrease marketing costs.

For these reasons, brand advocacy is 12 out of 10!!

BRANDING YOURSELF:
HOW TO DO SO IN FOUR EASY WAYS

If you're interested in branding your product or company, you may not be sure where to begin. The good news: I'm here to help. You can brand in many ways, but here I pare it down to four ways to help you start:

Branding by association

This way involves hanging out with and being seen with people who are very much higher than you in your particular niche.

Branding by achievement

This way repurposes your previous achievements.

Branding by testimonial

This way makes use of the testimonials that you receive but have likely never used.

Branding by WOW

A WOW is the pleasantly unexpected, the equivalent of going the extra mile. The easiest and most certain way to WOW people is to tell them that you've written a book. To discover how you can write a book of own, go to www.BrandingSmallBusinessForDummies.com.

25

Happiness:
How to Experience
the "Real Deals"

MARCI SHIMOFF

I was 41 years old, stretched out on a lounge chair by my pool and reflecting on my life. I had achieved all that I thought I needed to be happy.

You see, when I was a child, I thought there would be five main things that would ensure that I'd be happy: a successful career helping people, a loving husband, a comfortable home, a great body, and a wonderful circle of friends. After years of study, hard work, and a few "lucky breaks," I finally had them all. (Okay, so my body didn't quite look like Halle Berry's—but four out of five isn't bad!) You think I'd have been on the top of the world.

But surprisingly I wasn't. I felt an emptiness inside that the outer successes of life couldn't fill. I was also afraid that if I lost any of those things, I might be miserable. Sadly, I knew I wasn't alone in feeling this way.

While happiness is the one thing we all truly want, so few people really experience the deep and lasting fulfillment that fills our soul. Why aren't we finding it?

Because, in the words of the old country western song, we're looking for happiness in "all the wrong places."

Looking around, I saw that the happiest people I knew weren't the most successful and famous. Some were married, some were single. Some had lots of money, and some didn't have a dime. Some of them even had health challenges. From where I stood, there seemed to be no rhyme or reason to what made people happy. The obvious question became: *Could a person actually be happy for no reason?*

I had to find out.

So I threw myself into the study of happiness. I interviewed scores of scientists, as well as 100 unconditionally happy people. (I call them the Happy 100.) I delved into the research from the burgeoning field of positive psychology, the study of the positive traits that enable people to enjoy meaningful, fulfilling, and happy lives.

What I found changed my life. To share this knowledge with others, I wrote a book called *Happy for No Reason: 7 Steps to Being Happy from the Inside Out.*

One day, as I sat down to compile my findings, all the pieces of the puzzle fell into place. I had a simple, but profound "a-ha"—there's a continuum of happiness:

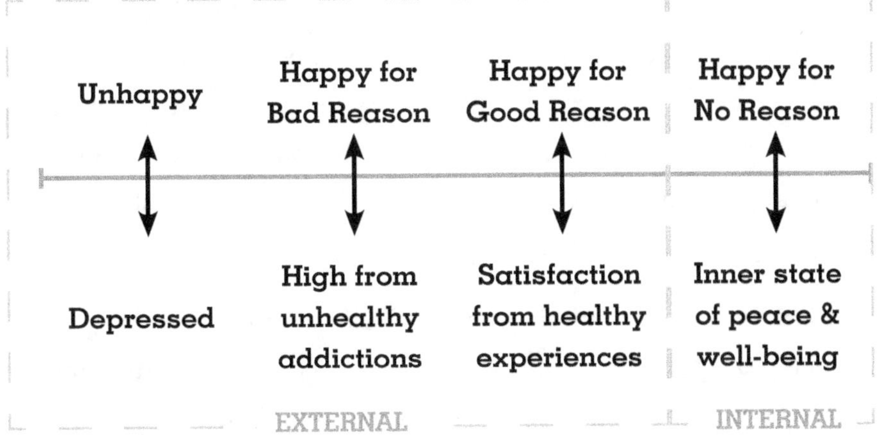

Unhappy: We all know what this means: life seems flat. Some of the signs are anxiety, fatigue, feeling blue or low—your "garden-variety" unhappiness. This isn't the same as clinical depression, which is characterized by deep despair and hopelessness that dramatically interferes with your ability to live a normal life, and for which professional help is absolutely necessary.

Happy for Bad Reason: When people are unhappy, they often try to make themselves feel better by indulging in addictions or behaviors that may feel good in the moment but are ultimately detrimental. They seek the highs that come from drugs, alcohol, excessive sex, "retail therapy," compulsive gambling, over-eating, and too much television-watching, to name a few. This kind of "happiness" is hardly happiness at all. It is only a temporary way to numb or escape our unhappiness through fleeting experiences of pleasure.

Happy for Good Reason: This is what people usually mean by happiness: having good relationships with our family and friends, success in our careers, financial security, a nice house or car, or using our talents and strengths well. It's the pleasure we derive from having the healthy things in our lives that we want.

Don't get me wrong. I'm all for this kind of happiness! It's just that it's only half the story. Being Happy for Good Reason depends on the external conditions of our lives—these conditions change or are lost, our happiness usually goes too. Relying solely on this type of happiness is where a lot of our fear is stemming from these days. We're afraid the things we think we need to be happy may be slipping from our grasp.

Deep inside, I think we all know that life isn't meant to be about getting by, numbing our pain, or having everything "under control." True happiness doesn't come from merely collecting an assortment of happy experiences. At our core, we know there's something more than this.

There is. It's the next level on the happiness continuum—Happy for No Reason.

Happy for No Reason: This is true happiness—a state of peace and well-being that isn't dependent on external circumstances.

Happy for No Reason isn't elation, euphoria, mood spikes, or peak experiences that don't last. It doesn't mean grinning like a fool 24/7 or experiencing a superficial high. Happy for No Reason isn't an emotion. In fact, when you are Happy for No Reason, you can have *any* emotion—including sadness, fear, anger or hurt—but you still experience that underlying state of peace and well-being.

When you're Happy for No Reason, you *bring* happiness to your outer experiences rather than trying to *extract* happiness from them. You don't need to manipulate the world around you to try to make yourself happy. You live from happiness, rather than *for* happiness.

This is a revolutionary concept. Most of us focus on being Happy for Good Reason, stringing together as many happy experiences as we can, like beads in a necklace, to create a happy life. We have to spend a lot of time and energy trying to find just the right beads so we can have a "happy necklace".

Being Happy for No Reason, in our necklace analogy, is like having a happy string. No matter what beads we put on our necklace—good, bad or indifferent—our inner experience, which is the string that runs through them all, is happy, and creates a happy life.

Happy for No Reason is a state that's been spoken of in virtually all spiritual and religious traditions throughout history. The concept is universal. In Buddhism, it is called causeless joy; in Christianity, the kingdom of Heaven within; and in Judaism it is called *ashrei*, an inner sense of holiness and health. In Islam it is called *falah*, happiness and well-being; and in Hinduism it is called *ananda*, or pure bliss. Some traditions refer to it as an enlightened or awakened state.

So how can you be Happy for No Reason?

Science is verifying the way. Researchers in the field of positive psychology have found that we each have a "happiness set-point," that determines our level of happiness. No matter what happens, whether it's something as exhilarating as winning the lottery or as challenging as a horrible accident, most people eventually return to their original happiness level. Like your weight set-point, which keeps the scale hovering around the same number, your happiness set-point will remain the same **unless you make a concerted effort to change it.** In the same way you'd crank up the thermostat to get comfortable on a chilly day, you actually have the power to reprogram your happiness set-point to a higher level of peace and well-being. The secret lies in practicing the habits of happiness.

Some books and programs will tell you that you can simply decide to be happy. They say just make up your mind to be happy—and you will be.

I don't agree.

You can't just decide to be happy, any more than you can decide to be fit or to be a great piano virtuoso and expect instant mastery. You can, however, decide to take the necessary steps, like exercising or taking piano lessons—and by practicing those skills, you can get in shape or give recitals. In the same way, you can become Happy for No Reason through practicing the habits of happy people.

All of your habitual thoughts and behaviors in the past have created specific neural pathways in the wiring in your brain, like grooves in a record. When we think or behave a certain way over and over, the neural pathway is strengthened and the groove becomes deeper—the way a well-traveled route through a field eventually becomes a clear-cut path. Unhappy people tend to have more negative neural pathways. This is why you can't just ignore the realities of your brain's wiring and *decide* to be happy! To raise your level of happiness, you have to create new grooves.

Scientists used to think that once a person reached adulthood, the brain was fairly well "set in stone" and there wasn't much you could do to change it. But new research is revealing exciting information about the brain's neuroplasticity: when you think, feel and act in different ways, the brain changes and actually rewires itself. You aren't doomed to the same negative neural pathways for your whole life. Leading brain researcher Dr. Richard Davidson, of the University of Wisconsin says, "Based on what we know of the plasticity of the brain, we can think of things like happiness and compassion as skills that are no different from learning to play a musical instrument or tennis …. it is possible to train our brains to be happy."

While a few of the Happy 100 I interviewed were born happy, most of them learned to be happy by practicing habits that supported their happiness. That means wherever you are on the happiness continuum, it's entirely in your power to raise your happiness level.

In the course of my research, I uncovered 21 core happiness habits that anyone can use to become happier and stay that way. You can find all 21 happiness habits at www.HappyForNoReason.com

Here are a few tips to get you started:

1. **Incline Your Mind Toward Joy.** Have you noticed that your mind tends to register the negative events in your life more than the positive? If you get ten compliments in a day and one criticism, what do you remember? For most people, it's the criticism. Scientists call this our "negativity bias" — our primitive survival wiring that causes us to pay more attention to the negative than the positive. To reverse this bias, get into the daily habit of consciously registering the positive around you: the sun on your skin, the taste of a favorite food, a smile or kind word from a co-worker or friend. Once you notice something positive, take a moment to savor it deeply and feel it; make it more than just a mental observation. Spend 20 seconds soaking up the happiness you feel.

2. **Let Love Lead.** One way to power up your heart's flow is by sending loving kindness to your friends and family, as well as strangers you pass on the street. Next time you're waiting for the elevator at work, stuck in a line at the store or caught up in traffic, send a silent wish to the people you see for their happiness, well-being, and health. Simply wishing others well switches on the "pump" in your own heart that generates love and creates a strong current of happiness.

3. **Lighten Your Load.** To make a habit of letting go of worries and negative thoughts, start by letting go on the physical level. Cultural anthropologist Angeles Arrien recommends giving or throwing away 27 items a day for nine days. This deceptively simple practice will help you break attachments that no longer serve you.

4. **Make Your Cells Happy.** Your brain contains a veritable pharmacopeia of natural happiness-enhancing neurochemicals — endorphins, serotonin, oxytocin, and dopamine — just waiting to be released to every organ and cell in your body. The way that you eat, move, rest, and even your facial expression can shift the balance of your body's feel-good-chemicals, or "Joy Juice", in your favor. To dispense some extra Joy Juice — smile. Scientists have discovered that smiling decreases stress hormones and boosts happiness chemicals, which increase the body's T-cells, reduce pain, and enhance relaxation. You may not feel like it, but smiling — even artificially to begin with — starts the ball rolling and will turn into a real smile in short order.

5. **Hang with the Happy.** We catch the emotions of those around us just like we catch their colds — it's called emotional contagion. So it's important to make wise choices about the company you keep. Create appropriate boundaries with emotional bullies and "happiness vampires" who suck the life out of you. Develop your happiness "dream team" — a mastermind or support group you meet with regularly to keep you steady on the path of raising your happiness.

"Happily ever after" isn't just for fairytales or for only the lucky few. Imagine experiencing inner peace and well-being as the backdrop for everything else in your life. When you're Happy for No Reason, it's not that your life always looks perfect — it's that, however it looks, you'll still be happy!

By Marci Shimoff. Based on the New York Times bestseller *Happy for No Reason: 7 Steps to Being Happy from the Inside Out*, which offers a revolutionary approach to experiencing deep and lasting happiness. The woman's face of the *Chicken Soup for the Soul* series and a featured teacher in *The Secret*, Marci is an authority on success, happiness, and the law of attraction. To order *Happy for No Reason* and receive free bonus gifts, go to www.happyfornoreason.com/mybook.

Sex, Love and Relationships

DR. JOHN GRAY

Just as great sex is important to lasting love, good health is important to sex and relationships. About 12 years ago, I cured myself of early stage Parkinson's disease. The doctors were amazed, but my wife was even more amazed. She noted that our relationship and sex life had become dramatically better. It turns out that the natural supplements I used to reverse Parkinson's can also make you more attentive and loving in your relationship. At that point, I realized that good relationship skills alone were not enough to sustain love and passion for a lifetime.

I shared many insights gained from my 40 years' experience as a marriage counselor and coach in *Men Are From Mars, Women Are From Venus*. And while my insights go a long way towards helping men and women understand and support each other, good communication skills alone are not always enough. For better relationships, we not only need to be healthy, but we must also experience optimum brain function.

If you are tired, depressed, anxious, not sleeping well, or in pain, then certainly romantic feelings will become a thing of the past. My recovery from Parkinson's revealed to me the profound connection between the quality of our health and our relationships. This insight has motivated me, over the past twelve years, to research the secrets of optimum health as a foundation for lasting love.

These are health secrets that are generally not explored in medical school. In medical school, doctors are indoctrinated into the culture of examining the symptoms, identifying the sickness, and prescribing a drug to treat that sickness. They learn very little about how to be healthy or to sustain successful relationships.

There are no university courses entitled "Better Nutrition For Better Sex". Drugs sometimes save lives, but they also have negative side effects that do little to preserve the passion in a relationship. Ideally, drugs should be used as a last resort and 90 % of our health plan should be drug free. From this perspective, the heath care crisis, as well as our high rate of divorce in America, is indirectly caused by our dependence on doctors and prescription drugs.

Most people have not even considered that taking prescribed drugs (even for the small stuff) can weaken their relationships, which in turn makes them more vulnerable to more disease. For example, if you are feeling depressed or anxious, a drug may numb your pain, but it does nothing to help you correct the cause of your problem. It can even prevent you from feeling your natural motivation to get the emotional support you need. In a variety of ways, our common health complaints are all expressions of two major conditions: our lack of education to identify and support unmet gender-specific emotional needs; and our lack of education to identify and support unmet gender-specific nutritional needs.

With an understanding of natural solutions that have been around for thousands of years, drugs are not needed to treat many common complaints. Some symptoms like low energy, weight gain, allergies, hormonal imbalance, mood swings, poor sleep, indigestion, lack of focus, ADD and ADHD, procrastination, low motivation, memory loss, decreased libido, PMS, vaginal dryness, muscle and joint pain, or the lack of passion in life and/or our relationships can be treated drug-free. By using drugs (even over-the-counter drugs) to treat these common complaints, our bodies and relationships are weakened, making us more vulnerable to bigger and more costly health challenges like cancer, diabetes, heart disease, auto-immune disease, dementia, and Alzheimer's. In simple terms, by handling the easy stuff (the common complaints) without doctors and drugs, we can protect ourselves from the big stuff (cancer, heart disease, dementia, etc.) We can be healthy and also enjoy lasting love and passion in our personal lives.

Even if you are taking anti-depressants or hormone replacement therapy, sometimes all it takes to stop treating the symptom is to directly handle the cause. With specific mineral orotates (something most people have never heard of) or omega three oil from the brains of salmon, your stress levels immediately drop and you begin to feel happy and in love again.

For every health challenge, we have explored the effects on our relationships, with as well as natural remedies that can sometimes produce immediate positive results. You can find these natural solutions to common health complaints for free at my website: www.MarsVenus.com.

What they don't teach in medical school is how to be healthy and happy without the use of drugs or hormone replacement. By refusing drugs and taking responsibility for your health, a wealth of new possibilities can become available to you. We are designed to be healthy and happy, and it is within our reach if we commit to increasing our knowledge.

New research regarding the brain differences in men and women reveals how specific nutritional supplements, combined with gender-specific relationship and self-nurturing skills, can stimulate the hormones of health, happiness and increased energy. Over the past 10 years in my healing center in California, I witnessed how natural solutions coupled with gender-specific relationship skills could solve our common health complaints without drugs. By addressing these common complaints without prescribed drugs, not only do we feel better, but our relationships have the potential to improve dramatically.

Ultimately the cause of all our common complaints is higher stress levels. Researchers around the world all agree that chronic stress levels in our bodies provide a basis for any and all disease to take hold. An easy and quick solution for lowering our stress reactions is specific nutritional support combined with gender-smart relationship skills. Extra nutritional support is needed because stress depletes the body very quickly of essential nutrients. When a car engine is running more quickly, it uses fuel more quickly. When we are stressed, we need both extra nutrients and extra emotional support. Understanding what we need to take and where to get it requires education. Every week day at www.MarsVenus.com I have a live daily show where I freely answer questions and provide this much-needed new gender-specific insight.

At www.MarsVenus.com, we are happy to share what we have learned for creating healthy bodies and positive relationships. You can find a host of natural solutions for common complaints and feel confident that you have the power to feel fully alive with an abundance of energy and positive feelings that will enrich all your relationships.

41

Break Through Your Barriers & Live Your Dreams

SANDRA WESTLAND

Every woman deserves to feel powerful and successful, and the opportunity to do so stands right before her. She doesn't have to be a warrior to smite every dragon or burn down every obstacle that stands in her way. She simply needs to connect with and be her real, authentic self. So her journey to success begins by standing still, by being curious about the world of potential that exists within her and in front of her, and by understanding her inner world in order to ignite change in her outer one towards her success.

But, what stops her from becoming the author of her own life, from being all she can be? The glass ceiling, the unofficial barrier that prevents women from rising up to executive positions or from running their successful businesses, does still exist. Yet, in my twenty-five years of education, hypnopsychotherapy and peak performance training, I see, more significantly, an individual's own inner glass ceiling capping and limiting the success in life that is there for the taking.

To be a woman is to be extraordinary. We all have it within us to move beyond an ordinary life and its everyday limitations to embrace our desires and possibilities, harness our untold natural potential and live the life we are meant to live —a life of personal freedom in which we simply are our natural, awesome selves. Your power is switched on when you embrace, embody, express and enjoy being a woman. Your energy is released when you learn to live truly in your own skin. I love being a woman, and I love continuing to find out just what that is like for me.

This is a journey of discovering your place in life as a woman and as a woman in business, a voyage into your inner mind's processing and the terrain of your inner world, deeper than your conscious mind can be aware of. It is an expedition through self-alignment, forming the detail of your desired outcomes, shaping your life to fit with your passions, sourcing the energy that drives you, thus smashing your glass ceiling and allowing your transformation to unfold. Just as I experienced my own first steps, I want you also to stride out along this path and the journey of becoming your potential. The message I write within the pages of *Smashing Your Glass Ceiling* takes you through this fascinating journey where "Wow, I didn't realize that" and "No wonder I wasn't getting to where I wanted to" are familiar insights.

HOW DOES IT ALL WORK?

The tools you will need for such a journey of self-discovery are drawn from Neuro-Linguistic Programming (NLP), guided imagery, and a gentle questing into uncovering your own uniqueness and meaning in life. In blending these time-tested methods into one programme, it's possible to break through all that's holding you back in life.

From my own personal experience as a woman and as a psychotherapist and trainer, I've found that one of the most powerful tools we naturally have and need to embrace first is the power of imagination; even if you think you have one or not, you really do have an amazing, creative imagination. It just may need awakening and a little encouraging. I would love to show you just how powerful your imagination can be and how crucial it is to connect with you and be your own woman. In beginning this imaginative journey, you are sparking off a chain of events that produce fundamental changes in your physical body, starting with the neurological processes that will link to your biology and produce within you "decision states" leading to the different outcomes that you want, easily and naturally. Imagine the decisions that you can make or the actions that you can take when you are feeling confident, in balance and aligned to your vision, compared to the choices that you opt for when you are upset, anxious, depressed and out of sync with yourself.

By guiding your imagination, you can form an internal vision in which you are taking the right path for you to succeed in your life, and then formulate just what that is. As you immerse yourself in the excitement and the thrill of being on the right road to greatness, you tap into the inner confidence and self-reliance, inner freedom and success awareness that generate your momentum to smashing your glass ceiling. The power is always within you. It's just a case of summoning and connecting with it.

Imagine also gaining new understanding into how you process information from your "now" experiences, how you view the world, how you communicate with others and how they communicate with you. Imagine how much easier your life would be. You can learn how to recognize ways of processing external data and how, by modifying your communication in a way that makes sense to others, your relationships become infinitely warmer, richer and more connected.

Think about meeting me in the flesh for the first time, already knowing how my inner world works. Wouldn't it be good to know I'm an auditory person? Why? Well, my world is very much filtered through sounds. I will be finely tuned into noise … all noise. I will get distracted with too much of it, and I will recognize very slight changes in your voice, tone and pitch. So I will hear a hint of doubt or an emotion rising from within you just by hearing your voice. If you speak too slowly or very loudly, this will create a dissonance within me. If you use language that talks about "viewing something" or "seeing what you mean" or "having a handle on this or that" instead of "sounds like" or "listen to", I will feel a mismatch between us. Don't click your pen or tap it on the table if you want me to be relaxed! It's only a slight inner discomfort, but it undeniably shapes how I experience you and your communication. Upon our meeting, if you appreciate my world and I appreciate yours, we will hit it off with ease. I will look to communicate to you through your world, which may be visual, auditory, kinesthetic or auditory digital, all very different ways of experiencing and processing, and you can do the same for me.

GETTING TO KNOW YOUR GLASS CEILING

Your internal glass ceiling may have been created from prejudgments, prejudices, cultural and social attitudes that operate deep within the unconscious, taken in when young. So, it's crucial to find these out and know how they work for you, to understand the inner conflicts that are holding you back and what they mean. In speaking with a senior executive upon her reading *Smashing Your Glass Ceiling*, she'd suddenly become aware of how she was dressing like a man for her banking boardroom meetings. It wasn't her at all, but after further exploration, she realized she had unconsciously thought it would help men relate to her and allow her to be "taken seriously". She was shocked at how unconscious this had been, but she was relieved to learn it and is now enjoying the fun of finding out who she is as a woman in business and what clothes this exploration leads her to wearing. It is only by excavating these unconscious gender biases and other judgments that contribute towards making your own ceiling that you can reveal your real, natural self to yourself and the world. In understanding yourself more and knowing just who you are and how you are in the world, you become free to choose how to respond to situations and to people, and then you really begin to own your own life.

I am wondering just what you are thinking, having read these thousand plus words. Is this possible for you or is your glass ceiling giving you bother, preventing you from imagining and thinking of all that you can be? What does your ceiling hold and what is it whispering to you right now? What is your "default" setting?

Are you someone who assumes you won't find a car parking space and prove yourself right, or do you simply know that it doesn't matter where you park and thus usually find one just when and where you need it? Is a potential redundancy at work a chance to do something different, or a terrible catastrophe that you will never escape? Your attitudes play a massive part in your life experiences, and to how much you can grow. Zig Ziglar's famous saying "Your attitude determines your altitude" is so true. So, how do your attitudes determine how successful you can be?

I have lived and refined through my own personal journey a framework of all the things that are crucial to help you aspire to be. Let's make a start right now, something to get you thinking. Let's peek into those achieving just what you want and begin to emulate some of what they do and how they are. It's as good a place as any to start!

In NLP terms, this is called "modeling". In modeling the behaviors and habits of successful people, we're seeking to learn from successful businesswomen and successful women just what it is that they do, and what it is that they have that makes them successful; not to become them, but to incorporate their winning behaviours into our repertoire, choosing those which are congruent with us and amplifying them. I often explore other women that I admire and am drawn to. In carefully watching what they do and exploring this within my own life, in my way, I can open up to further resources that I naturally have, but have yet to connect with. In Sue Knight's' words, "If you spot it, you've got it." (NLP at Work, 2013)

Now to stoke up those neurological pathways as we vamp it up a little more and transport you forward into your own fabulous future. Familiarize yourself with the state of being successful with no glass ceiling, as if you've already accomplished that level of success, a dress rehearsal if you like. Put on the mantle of success and ask yourself how and what do you feel, how would your day evolve, what can you do now that you couldn't do before. How would others perceive you? Get your brain to make it a done deal so that it can look for it, search it out and create it. This is the self-fulfilling prophecy at its most positive, potent and powerful.

Anticipate now becoming friendly and familiar with a future you who has everything you need and want and to be able to use the guidance of that future you – the answers may very well surprise you. My future self enlightened me as to my fear of success! This helped me find my inner glass ceiling and the meaning of it all, so I could smash it and really begin to find out just what I could do and what was possible in life. I believe that to guide others you have to have lived the journey yourself, and so my own personal journey has and is this path too, encompassing where I am finding myself … as a woman, an educator, therapist and businesswoman. This is a journey I don't ever intend to stop.

PEELING BACK THE ONION

There is so much more to explore! As humans, we've infinite depths, so exploring your inner beliefs, your values and mission is crucial for success. It's the peeling back of the onion, layer by layer (corny, I know), but I assure you that the exploration, while deep, is richly rewarding. Wouldn't you rather know what's holding you back and why you may feel frustrated with yourself? I know I would. I simply want to make the most of my time on this earth and experience it as much as possible. Life is to be lived and not simply endured and got through.

Excavate your inner beliefs, isolate the limiting ones that have held you back, and then you will easily and naturally begin to fly! Once figured out, you become empowered as you re-think and re-frame beliefs into being resourceful, productive and desirable, and turn them into second nature.

Let's go one deeper. Do you know just what it is that you value, all those things that are really important to you? Are they aligned with your life? These are your GPS, and if you're frustrated, feel trapped in the mundane of life or have unwanted physical/emotional symptoms, then value fine-tuning is needed for you to move forward in the direction that you want to go. Let's not be sidetracked by detours, road closures and an unclear destination. Being authentic and all that you are needs you to know what you value so that you're able to craft your mission for the ultimate alignment. In *Smashing Your Glass Ceiling* or my Success workshops , you will not short-change yourself here. I will journey with you, helping you along the way through a process of simple, yet profoundly powerful steps.

When you are fully aligned, there will be no holding you back. You'll meet the right person at the right time, and you'll have the right skills to achieve your goals. Everything will fall into place like a jigsaw puzzle, and you'll have "the strength, the patience, and the passion to reach for the stars", to borrow the words of a courageously inspiring woman, Harriet Tubman.

LOADING UP ON INTERNAL RESOURCES

It's not all plain sailing, and you *will* be derailed by the unexpected, but what makes someone a success is their ability to keep going, even when challenged. So, one of the final steps in the Programme is to load you up with the internal resources to get you through when things get sticky, and when, quite frankly, you wonder why you bother. NLP strategies reprogram how we react and respond to such times, making a monumental difference to how you experience your life. If you're feeling down on yourself, I will show you that you can change your physiology. If you're getting increasingly anxious about an upcoming meeting, you can change your self-talk, the inner conversation you're having with yourself, to something more upbeat, more encouraging and more positive.

Powerful NLP strategies are there for you to use at any time and in any situation. Your life will be richer and filled with more options when you are able to redirect your thinking and focus, stay resourceful in stressful situations, and generate behaviors and outcomes that are positive for you and your life.

Finally, if this chapter has inspired you to delve deeper into Smashing your Glass Ceiling, the book comes with a number of bonuses, some of which can be downloaded from my website, www.SmashingYourGlassCeiling.com for you to enjoy absolutely free. So, get started now and embrace the fact that you are an extraordinary woman.

TAKING THE FIRST STEP

All of us have to start somewhere. I did when I was thirty-four, when I found myself looking at twenty-six more years before retirement, counting the years and the days till the next school holiday. Not how I imagined my life would be.

By becoming curious, asking questions of myself and tapping into effective life-changing techniques that opened me up to the power and potential of the mind, I'm on a fascinating journey. I'm continuing to smash my own internal glass ceiling, and am living out my passion to enhance the lives of other women. I am certainly not "sorted out", nor have I "self-actualized" and not every day is "grrreat", but I know that every day is an adventure with the chance to grow further and find out more about just what is possible.

The more women I meet and work with, the more I learn and the more I gather evidence to support my belief that, as women, we owe it to ourselves to be extraordinary. This is my invitation to you to take the first steps with me on your own journey of becoming all you wish to be.

Sandra Westland is an experienced educator, therapist and successful businesswoman who helps others to find their passion and fulfil their dreams. She has a Master's degree in Existential Psychotherapy, an Education Honours degree, and is a practicing Advanced Hypnotherapist and NLP practitioner. Her doctoral thesis explores women and their relationship with their bodies. She is the author of Smash Your Glass Ceiling and co-author of Thinking Therapeutically.

Sandra is a Director of the Contemporary College of Therapeutic Studies, where she trains people at life changing junctures to be aspiring therapists, so they too can enjoy the enriching privilege of helping others to find their path in life. She is also a co-founder of Self Help School™, which provides psycho-education for the public and is an international speaker on the power of the mind for change.

Enter Into a Passionate Relationship with Your Own Life

SILVANA L. AVRAM

Have you ever wondered whether there is more to life than meets the eye? Do you feel that despite all your achievements true fulfilment still eludes you?

Join me on this transformational journey where you will learn to see yourself and your life in a different light.

- You will find out how to ask the right questions.

- You will learn to identify the main reason why you find yourself trapped in the same vicious circle.

- You will redefine the true meaning of being and uncover the source of deep fulfilment.

- You will be able to decide whether you are ready to embark on the journey to personal fulfilment.

My passionate plea to you is to allow this introduction to the secret of lasting fulfilment to work as a powerful catalyst for you. Should you want to explore the topics addressed here in more depth I invite you to read my book "Being You And Loving You – The Ultimate Guide To Fulfilment" – where I guide you through twelve life changing steps to true fulfilment. Together with the book you will also find plenty of free materials, insights and support at www.BeingYouAndLovingYou.com

It is the aim of this chapter to empower you to start your journey to true fulfilment. Are you ready? Let's dive in!

YOUR JOURNEY TO FULFILMENT STARTS WITH ASKING THE RIGHT QUESTIONS

"The Universe contains three things that cannot be destroyed;
Being, Awareness and LOVE"

— Deepak Chopra

"What is the meaning of life?" Human beings have searched for an answer to this question for millennia. Sages, philosophers, religious figures and scientists have all put forward their hypotheses, and each interpretation added yet another nuance to a mystery that remains as fascinating and as alluring as it has always been.

So: "Why are we here?" And why is it that this most important question of all is also one of the most avoided? Perhaps we have long accepted that there is no answer to it. Perhaps facing this question feels so…unsettling that we prefer to bury it under more…urgent matters. Like finding a job and paying the next bill.

I put to you another possibility. I believe that "Why are we here?" is indeed an unanswerable question. At least for the time being. And so is *"What is the meaning of life?"*

Why? Because they are too vast…and too vague!

Does that mean I am advising you to drop the questioning altogether and simply get on with your life? No, not at all! Not if you want to live a joyous, meaningful life. Not if you are looking for true fulfilment. In fact, if this is what you are after, it is vitally important to keep questioning.

But you must learn to ask the right questions.

I believe that each one of us must start with the more manageable "Why *am I* here?" or "What is the meaning of *my* life?"

I believe that each one of us must take responsibility for our own answers.

You see, when you allow someone else to answer these questions for you, you give away your power (and with that your responsibility). You may like a particular answer/ philosophy for a while and you may find it resonates with you – you may even dedicate your life to promoting it – but it will still not be yours – and as such it will not fully transform your life, it will not bring you the fulfilment you crave. You may read as many books as you want and you may attend endless wonderful seminars…They will all help you feel good for a while and you are sure to get some valuable insight. But no person and no book can truly change your life for you. Only when you find the strength and the courage to stay with the question of meaning long enough to allow for your own answer to be born in you, will you find the infinite joy and freedom that come from knowing. It is only *your own* answer that will truly transform *your life*. It is owning that answer that brings true fulfilment.

If your life is a riddle, the only way to fully - fill it… is to find your own answer to it.

Now that you know where to start…how do you actually do it?

You can find your own answer by asking the right questions, either on your own or by engaging in a philosophical dialogue with friends and other people interested in the same quest for meaning. You must be patient and tenacious, and not give up at the first signs of exhaustion or disappointment. After all, the question of meaning is the most challenging question of all, and many choose to avoid it altogether. But if you stay with it, if you make it an intrinsic part of your journey, sooner or later you will be rewarded.

You will not be alone in your endeavour. One of the most famous of the Delphic maxims inscribed in the pronaos (forecourt) of the Temple of Apollo at Delphi, Ancient Greece, and quoted by many, most famously by Socrates as the main character in Plato's dialogues, was *"Know Thyself"*. Through the ages there have been many who have embarked on this arduous journey.

Today, there is a modern variant of the life-transforming dialogues left to posterity by Plato: the coaching dialogue. The Philosopher is replaced by the more modest Coach. They are similar, however, in that the Coach, like the Greek philosopher but unlike a religious figure or a mentor, is not providing the answers. Instead, she or he is merely providing you with the right questions, gently challenging you when you go off track and often holding a symbolic mirror in which you start to see your true reflection and find your own answers.

It is a true measure of our 21st Century's *Age of Knowledge* that Coaching has become such an accessible experience. Perhaps this is a sign that more and more amongst us are ready and willing to stay with the question of meaning and find the true purpose of our lives. Perhaps more and more people are ready to embark on the journey to true fulfilment. Are you?

BEING SUCCESSFUL IS NOT THE SAME AS SUCCEEDING AT BEING

"What makes you think human beings are sentient and aware? There's no evidence for it. Human beings never think for themselves, they find it too uncomfortable. For the most part, members of our species simply repeat what they are told – and become upset if they are exposed to any different view. The characteristic human trait is not awareness but conformity.."

— Michael Crichton

"I am a human being, not a human doing. Don't equate your self-worth with how well you do things in life. You aren't what you do. If you are what you do, then when you don't...you aren't."

— Dr. Wayne Dyer

Before we proceed to consider what your journey to true fulfilment might look like when you embark on a path of enquiry and examination, I would like you to briefly stop and take a look at your life right now.

Do you love your life? Do you love yourself? Do you feel deep gratitude and awe about who you are? Do you feel blissful, fulfilled and radiant, sharing your wisdom and your light with everyone else, in compassion?

Chances are that you don't.

Chances are that you don't even believe this is possible!!

But if it were possible, would you like to feel like this? Would you like to live your life with absolute joy, and share your happiness with others?

I hope your answer to that last question is yes.

If it is, you have already taken the first step to fulfilment.

You see, most people have already given up on personal fulfilment. Most people have somehow fallen into the trap of believing that there is nothing more to life than work, duty, supporting family and friends, and the occasional recreation. It may sound incredible, but most people have convinced themselves that life is more about sacrifice and suffering than about being happy. If asked, of course everyone would say they want to be happy. Yet most people spend their lives doing things that take them farther and farther away from being joyful and fulfilled.

Most people spend most of their lives *doing* things. In fact doing so many things that they don't have the time to stop and ask *why* they are doing them.

Most people spend their lives doing so many things that they forget to Be.

But how can I forget to be? I hear you ask.

What else is there to 'being' that I haven't got already? Is it not enough that I am…alive? How can I be …being? How can I Be more?

You see…rocks and trees and animals are too. They exist. Life flows through them and expresses through them without encountering much opposition. They are pure expressions of life.

And so are we. Except for the fact that we also have the wonderful gifts of thought, of mind…of consciousness.

I want you to consider that maybe, just maybe, for us humans it is not enough to be alive, to truly Be. If it were, we would all be happy – or at least at ease. We would not ask questions. We would not search for more.

What makes us different is that we have the gift of being able to be aware of being. It is this gift, and whether or not we choose to use it, that makes all the difference.

In order to truly Be as a human being you must be aware of who you are – of your potential. You must get involved in "being", become responsible for your "being", become the co-creator of your life.

When, on the other hand, we choose not to use the gift of awareness, we spend most of our lives doing things, being alive without truly being aware of the mystery, the complexity and the beauty of our being. We allow doing to take over, we throw ourselves into doing with a vengeance, seeking solace in temporary achievements that often leave us emptier than before.

Why and how does this happen? When we live without fully being present to our own lives, to our own being, we function on automatic pilot much of the time. Most of the functions we perform require so little of our conscious input that we get used to being disengaged. It's easier. We do the minimum and we get by. If we are "lucky" we can spend our whole life without having to account for the huge lack of …presence in it. For the most part, everyone is doing the same, and we are covered. No one will know. No one will dare ask.

But is that truly "lucky"? Is our life really about "getting by"?

If it were, mere survival would qualify as fulfilment. You would already and at all times feel fulfilled. Yet most of us know deep down inside our hearts that our lives must be more than just survival.

Perhaps our life is about success?

The difference between success and fulfilment is that success, as it tends to be defined, is still at the level of doing. You can become successful by following instructions and still staying on autopilot. In fact, the more autopilot-friendly the system you follow, the more successful you probably are in that particular area.

It is a common mistake to equate success with fulfilment. Many people who do, realize that success has not brought them the fulfilment they wished for. Many of these people spend years wondering where they went wrong and what's missing.

Our society seems to conspire to push us towards a narrowly defined form of success that rarely allows any space for true fulfilment. In other words, our misinterpretations are not entirely our fault. We are taught from early on to play by the (widely accepted) rules. We trust our parents and our teachers, and we unwittingly follow in their footsteps. We keep ourselves busy doing so many things that we have little time for self-exploration or personal inquiry, for Being. It is this restless drive for doing more and more that slowly but surely derails us from the only achievement that matters: understanding, accepting and expressing – in fact Being - our true self. Unless we stop to ask the right questions we don't even realise what we are missing.

To sum it up, success in doing cannot lead to fulfilment, for the simple reason that it involves operating at a different level.

To achieve true fulfilment you must operate at the level of Being.

It is not being successful at doing that will make you feel fulfilled.

To be fulfilled you must succeed at Being.

* * * *

So far we have learnt that in order to be fulfilled you must start by asking the right questions: "What is the meaning of my life?" "Why am I here?"

Tackling these and similar questions of meaning helps you become aware: aware that there is more to life than meets the eye; aware that as a human being it is not enough to be alive…Nor is it enough to be doing many things.

We then looked at what happens when you don't ask these questions. When you avoid questioning the true meaning of your life you get sucked into a life of endless doing with very little time for Being – and hence, with very little or no chance of feeling fulfilled.

For most people the question of meaning is an intimidating one, and one they'd rather put aside. After all, why take responsibility for one's life when it seems easier to just get by? Many people "succeed" in avoiding this question altogether. They also miss the opportunity of living deeply fulfilling, joyful lives. For others, something happens that forces them to wake up to it. It could be an unexpected turn of fate, a tragic event, even a major bonus, like winning the lottery, that pushes them to take a deeper look in the mirror. At those times they discover that there is a whole new dimension to 'being' that they were completely ignoring before. It is then up to them to embark on a journey of discovery that should ultimately lead them to true fulfilment.

There is, of course, a more natural, organic way that comes when you simply decide to take responsibility for your life and actively explore the gifts it promises to offer. You do it because you realize this is the only way you are going to feel truly happy and fulfilled. You do it because you want to be a co –creator in your life and express your full potential.

Along the way you may need the help of a friend, a sage or a coach – and you may be able to help others – but ultimately each one of us must find our own answers in order to express the true richness of our lives.

Once you are on the path to fulfilment there is no going back. You taste the ecstasy of being alive. Everything thereafter is a miraculous discovery, a wonderful adventure, a self-affirming deed and a deeply fulfilling expression of who you are. You have been kissed by life.

TRUE FULFILMENT COMES FROM AN AUTHENTIC AND LOVING RELATIONSHIP WITH YOUR LIFE

"The first step toward change is awareness. The second step is acceptance."

— Nathaniel Branden

We have established that in order to find true fulfilment you must be able to start with the right question and you must be able and willing to stay with it until you find your own answer. This is no easy journey. But it is the only one that will get you to true fulfilment. And as such, it is the most exciting journey of all.

If you are looking for deeper fulfilment, if you have started to realise that fulfilment will not come from doing more "stuff", chances are that you are already awakening to the possibility of an infinitely richer you. It does not matter how long it took you to get to this point. What matters is that you are ready: ready to embark on the beautiful, empowering, liberating and ultimately fulfilling journey of Being; ready to Be. Now.

Congratulations! Let the journey begin!

* * * *

As a coach, I can never get tired of seeing my clients find true joy and meaning in their lives. It often feels as if I watch them learn how to fly. And when they take off on their own…The sense of unlimited potential, freedom and happiness that comes with finding your own answer to the mystery of life is truly indescribable. One must experience it to be able to understand it.

But, if you will allow me, I would like to share with you what you might expect along the way.

There are two essential ingredients that will ensure a successful journey.

1.   In order to be fulfilled you must first learn to Be.

2.   Then you must learn how to Love Being.

As we touched upon earlier, truly Being requires presence and awareness.

True fulfilment comes when you and your life become one. When you live passionately…fully. To be one with life you must first wake up to Being; you must be aware of who you really are.

To start with, this will involve exploring your strengths, your talents, your gifts. It will mean looking at what makes you *you*, what makes you unique. In case you are already backing off in fear, rest assured. Every one of us is unique. Your special features, your memories and stories, your thoughts and feelings, your desires and dreams…all these make you a world unto itself, a uniquely beautiful expression of life, an exquisite original work of art in constant motion. There is no one else in the entire universe like you. There has never been and there will never be! You just have to muster the courage to embrace this truth! And allow it to transform you! It will help to have someone else hold the mirror, but once you learn to look at yourself in this way you will be able to see your life in a different light.

(To learn more about how you can embrace and celebrate your uniqueness visit www.BeingYouAndLovingYou.com)

It will then be important to find ways to truly express who you are; to listen to your heart and let it teach you everything you had tried to forget. Becoming aware of your thought patterns and connecting with your deepest emotions will enable you to re-define yourself. Then you can move one step further and try your hand at re-creating who you are. Being you is the gift you were given. Accepting this gift and then bettering it will be the gift you give back to life. How wonderful. This is pure creation. It's a miraculous process. Let it be fun!

At this point you should be ready to start thinking of how you could share your gift with others. This will become your purpose. That's when the real magic begins. And with it, true joy.

This is the point on your journey when your love relationship with life truly begins. The intimate loving relationship that you have managed to build with yourself expands into a passionate love affair with your life.

Now that you have become the co-creator of your life you must allow yourself to fall in love with your creation. You and your life must become one. This means moving from living your life into allowing your life to live, to express through you. You must be in awe of your life, you must respect it and cherish it and place it above anything else. Because your life is your gift to yourself and to the world. Because your life is the most intimate expression of who you are.

Loving your life is acknowledging and loving the infinite potential that you are. Loving your life with passion will teach you how to love every life with passion – will help you connect with every other life in compassion and joy. Knowing that you have expressed the best of you gives you the licence to feel free, to feel happy, to feel fulfilled.

When you live your life with this intensity there is a point where you will have to lose yourself to find yourself. That is when you must confront your deepest fear. Just as you have learnt to love yourself you must prepare to lose yourself. This is your ultimate act of sacrifice. You understand that your life does not belong to you. And this makes you love it even more. Now living your best possible life truly becomes your mission – and the only measurement of feeling true fulfilment.

You are now close, very close in fact, to fulfilment. You have already had glimpses of it – and you have started to feel its presence more and more poignantly. It is a mysterious, evasive feeling but one that is constant, and constantly making you blush. It permeates your life like a subtle perfume, like the light filling a room – like the presence of joy.

Your wonderful ability to be has now become a living example for others to see. By being you and fulfilling your mission you gift the world with your presence, and your life is the very proof of your fulfilment.

You inspire, you touch other lives and you share your wisdom and your joyful awareness with ease.

You live your life with the profound and blissful awareness of having achieved true fulfilment and the immense gratitude of having been able to do so.

* * * *

How does that feel? I hope you were able to get a glimpse of what it might mean to walk the journey to fulfilment. Often the transformation that takes place is difficult to put into words.

Suffice it to say that in this magical process you and your life will be completely transformed.

You enter a true partnership with life. You fall in love with your life and you become a co-creator of your life. That is the true meaning of being one with life. You live passionately – vibrantly. You express through your life and your life expresses through you.

To love being, to be in love with your life, is to step beyond being you into the miraculous field of living your life in service to Life – of giving your life as a gift back to Life. Everything you do at this level enriches you and enhances your life while affirming Life itself.

True fulfilment comes from being authentic and accomplishing your potential – thus fulfilling and honouring the unique opportunity that your life is.

(Explore more and get inspired with the wealth of insights and materials on the topic of being you, loving you and transcending you…that you will find at: www.BeingYouAndLovingYou.com)

LIVING A FULFILLING LIFE: IF NOT NOW, WHEN?

"Waking up is not a selfish pursuit of happiness, it is a revolutionary stance, from the inside out, for the benefit of all beings in existence."

– Noah Levine

We have explored together what it takes to embark on the journey to personal fulfilment.

We saw that it all starts with asking the right questions. We looked at what might happen when we fail to ask these questions. Then we had a glimpse at what to expect once we embark on this journey. I suppose the only question left is…Are you in?

You see… You either are or you aren't feeling fulfilled right now. And if you aren't, you are faced with a serious choice. True personal fulfilment involves presence and passion. You can't tell your life "I will live you tomorrow" or "I will love you tomorrow." You can't tell your mission, your purpose "I will be with you later." You have to be ready, open to it now. You have to commit to living your best possible life now.

The journey to fulfilment is not the easiest. It does require courage, honesty, a deep sense of wonder, the desire to overcome fears and the capacity to accept life's ephemeral and mysterious nature – and love it all the more for it.

To truly know fulfilment you must make the transition from living at the doing level to living at the Being level. Being successful has nothing to do with being fulfilled. Succeeding at Being has everything to do with it.

To truly succeed at Being you must go on a journey of self-discovery, and learn to celebrate your uniqueness, your richness, your unique expression, your feelings. You must learn to become a conscious co-creator of your life and then find the best ways to share your creation.

With this you move towards learning to love yourself and falling in love with your life. Once you learn to love yourself you must overcome your fear of losing yourself. This gives you the freedom to share yourself with the world.

By doing this you become an inspiration to others. You share the light of awareness with others. Finally you give back your life to Life with and for others – and in this you find ultimate fulfilment.

I don't know of a more wondrous journey – or one that is more worth it. You have been invited. The door has been opened for you. But only you can walk this journey and make your life the most extraordinary adventure of all. It is your life. Will you make it your fulfilment?

FINAL THOUGHT

If these pages have inspired you, you are probably ready to embark on the journey to fulfilment. Sometimes all we need is for someone to point the way. At other times we need someone to hold our hand as we learn how to fly on our own. I believe that Coaching can do that.

I believe that we live in a world where holding hands and learning from each other is soon becoming the norm. It is the only way in which we will be able to move forward. It is the only way in which we will learn, together, to truly Be. To be in love with our lives and to honour our potential. To find deep and lasting fulfilment. To share our richness and our beauty with everyone else, in joy. You can do it! See you there!

* * * *

Silvana is a successful Inspirational Coach, philosopher, writer and teacher.

More than anything else Silvana is a passionate human being driven by a deep commitment to create a better, happier world for everyone. She founded Life Coaching with Silvana to reach out and make her own contribution through empowering individuals to embrace and fulfil their potential, follow their dreams and live life with joy and gratitude. Silvana currently lives in the UK and divides her time between writing, coaching, group coaching, teaching, travelling, supporting humanitarian projects and conducting workshops and seminars.

To get in touch with Silvana, to know more about her Coaching practice, her projects and the events she organizes visit www.LifeCoachingWithSilvana.com

To get her book "Being You and Loving You – The Ultimate Guide To Fulfilment" together with free materials and more insights into the topic of fulfilment visit: www.BeingYouAndLovingYou.com

Honor Your Inner Treasures

CELINA TIO

COLLECTIVE CREATED ME

"We are all created from our experiences, and the first step towards embracing our inner treasures is to acknowledge this. You are wonderful, and the experiences that took you to this point are all part of that. Do not be afraid of yourself; instead, let yourself shine." This quote is from my recent book, *Honor Your Inner Treasures*. It's an underlying principle of that work, and its message is most certainly applicable to what you're about to read in this chapter of *The Authorities*. Collective Created Me explains in the *Honor Your Inner Treasures* book, how most of our beliefs are obtained through training and repetition, and assumed personality through education. Becoming aware of the Collective Created Me is extremely beneficial because it puts you on the road to self-acceptance and realization, forgiveness, independence, appreciation and true happiness.

Think about this for a moment: do you remember someone in your family being sick when you were a child? Were the hours spent in family time talking about symptoms, where pain started, where it ended, how long it lasted, and medicines? It's likely that much of the conversation also revolved around nurses, doctors' assessments and trips to the hospital. Soon, with so much health and sickness related information taken in, you unconsciously started to become so familiar enough with that illness that you accepted it as just part of your family. It became so normal that you could quickly respond to questions about it as if it were your illness, too. "My uncle Charlie had it, and so did his son and my grandmother. It runs in our family."

Imagine if the conversation you heard about Uncle Charlie's illness had been about the way that healthy habits, physical activities, and letting go of toxic thoughts helped him recover. What would you have learned to do then in the event of an illness?

This example of negativity changing your perspective is applicable to other life experiences. What about love and relationships? Conversations about unfaithfulness, divorce, unhealthy relationships, abuse, violence? How has the negativity of those conversations affected your beliefs and the actions you've taken in life? Money is another example. People often say they never have enough money. Stories are shared about someone's new business failing, or friends who've lost their homes because they couldn't make their mortgage payments. Wouldn't stories of success have a more positive impact to encourage others to improve in their lives?

Most people receive diagnoses during their lives pertaining to health, personal finances, the country's economy, beauty, fashion and relationships. Usually, these diagnoses are fully accepted as truth and fact. There is an alternative, however. Why not see a diagnosis as feedback of that exact, precise moment and utilize it as the moment of opportunity to change, to create, to expand, to become, to discover, is opening up for you?

People often say when a door closes a window opens, and wait for the window to open right in front of them. Often, hoping that the window will magically pop open and the situation will change. The sad thing is, it may take a while and in the meantime the beliefs that life is not fair, life is hard or life is good to others start to run your thoughts.

I want you to know that all windows and doors are always open for you. Even more, there are no windows, there are no doors, because once you embrace your greatness you are free to live with purpose.

Going back to our example of listening to other people's life experiences, can you perceive how your fears and beliefs originated during these events? The occasions are wonderful moments to enjoy and remember the past, but sometimes people retell stories about illnesses with as much detail as they can recall. It's possible the now-adult children have no recollection of the event's seriousness because they remember with a child's naïveté only how happy they were about recovery. Now, listening to the story of an experience in your life that evoked sadness, these adults inevitably feel pulled down and relive that low-energy feeling. You can change that feeling in you and all the people around you. Next time you are at a reunion be sure to evoke moments that bring joy and laughter. Everyone will leave feeling great, having enjoyed the party, and with a more positive attitude for the next adventure in their life.

BECOME AWARE - CONNECT WITH YOUR INNER BEING

Let go of the stories and let go of others' experiences. Start living your own.

Embrace the belief that your life is complete and absolute just as is. Take a deep breath, aware of your body, starting at the top and working your way down. Begin with your scalp, your hair, your temples, your forehead, your eyebrows, your eyes, then move on until you reach the tip of your toes. It's important to take in every part of yourself so don't stop at the surface. Recognize your organs and their functions, even noting your breath as it travels into your lungs and fills you with pure oxygen. Become aware of your being. I ask that you become aware of your being, not that you look into the mirror or take a selfie and analyze it to see if you have wrinkles, or criticize your body shape. Stop judging yourself and start knowing yourself.

Selfies have become, to many, a tool to prove oneself, or a tool of confirmation of existence, presence and self-acceptance, and others' approval of the moment that is being lived.

As if the moment being lived needs external approval to be considered as a "perfect moment" and only then sharing it with the world.

When you look at the moment you are living as an image that "looks good" or "like happiness", the gap between what you are doing "looks great", and truly feeling great, is large. There is no enjoyment or happiness if it always depends on others' opinions. Making a picture look good when the emotions you are feeling at the moment don't match the illusion of the created image is keeping you from living a true honest happy moment.

Different from this is taking a picture to capture a moment of real pleasure and happiness, and the peace and joy that healthy relationships and celebrations bring. Those are photographs that recall true emotions of happiness, in turn aligning your whole being into feeling truly amazing. These selfies are not only a moment taken with a camera; they are taken into your soul, leaving a long-lasting impression in your life. Those are moments that you will truly love to share with others without deleting anything. What is your selfie telling you when you look at it? What is that image revealing?

Become aware of yourself and the moment without editing. Be completely honest about everything. In this moment of self-awareness, accept everything – your age, aches, sadness, longings, best memories, dreams – without shyness, even if they look too big at this moment. Become aware because for the first time in your life you will be truly, honestly and entirely present with yourself, as you know yourself to be at this moment. What is your inner self telling you? This is the true SELF you should be contemplating.

If you do this, for the first time in your life you will be truly, honestly and entirely present. Your unique, true self will be revealed. For many people, doing this will be the scariest meeting of their lives. To me it is the most amazing!

When working with my clients, this point of their journey is the most exciting to me. As their guide to reaching their true inner being throughout the Honor Your Inner Treasures™ Program, the transformation the client undergoes is magical, because their life suddenly expands as they embrace and accept fully their inner self.

YOUR EMOTIONS ARE POWERFUL. LEARN FROM THEM.

Pretending is the only sure thing someone does when they are denied their true feelings. Pretending to feel well, smiling just with the movement of the facial muscles, repeating clichés as a consolation to true feelings, and distancing ourselves from loved ones or hiding from life aren't effective measures. Not talking about problems doesn't solve them. On the contrary, the repetition of those actions and inner messages undoubtedly becomes the reality in your life, which extends the sadness, insecurity, lack of confidence, and low-energy life. It's an unhealthy cycle, difficult to break. Have you ever heard people complaining about the good luck of others, or blaming the sad circumstances in their life on other people's lives? If you come close to a person behaving this way, stay away. You don't want to adopt that attitude.

You can change, you can become more, and you can be the best amazing you because you truly, genuinely feel it. Sharing your life with others with honesty, because there is absolutely nothing to hide, is liberating. Accept that you are a human being experiencing life, and in the process are growing, becoming, expanding, and evolving.

Through this process there will be moments that call for change, whether of habits, beliefs, actions, or behaviors. Change is a process of evolving into a different state. The emotions that you carry through the transition are of most importance. Are you making the change out of resentment or fear? Is it happening because you don't feel you're enough? Or are you just resigning yourself because you are obedient to unhappiness. What if you make the change because you know that you would love and enjoy doing something different?

Ask yourself what you need to make this change? Maybe it's taking a course or learning something new. Going through training is a fun ride when all you are doing is acquiring new skills to master what you love to do! Don't let the fear of change keep you from becoming healthier and happier. You look and feel healthy and beautiful when you are enjoying the moments that you are creating in your life. Change gives you jolts of energy that propels you to do more.

CHANGE TO THE POSITIVE SIDE OF LIFE

"Change the thinking positive and acting negative attitude." – Celina Tio

I hear people talking about difficult situations in their lives that end with usual comments like "I'm staying positive," "I'm trying to think positive" or "Hopefully…" However, simply repeating the mantra "I'm staying positive" does not make it true. When you are vibrating in the true sense of positive energy your life has no room for negative energy. Positive will always see, hear, understand, interpret, and plan in a constructive manner. When clients come for their first consultations with me, I listen attentively to their voices. From their tones I can hear the negative energy of unhealed wounds, regardless of the words they use. They tell their stories as if they've become comfortable hurting. This is a common means of self-defense and emotional survival.

In their journeys through the Honor Your Inner Treasures™ Program, clients delve into their true selves and are guided through the process of transmuting their thoughts into a positive perspective. This transformation occurs once we do the necessary inner work at the soul level, which is the purest essence of being. Anger may become understanding and compassion; resentment an opportunity for self-reflection and inner growth; and solitude a time of self-forgiveness and self-acceptance. The more you discover about your inner being, the closer you are to the positive energy of your true self. Knowing that each step my clients take brings them closer to their inner being of positive creation gives me great joy. It is important to create life experiences in such a way that, when you reflect on the past, all you see is a magical garden of your own design that you can be proud of having imagined, lived, grown and created.

Let's do an exercise that will assist you with looking at decisions based on fear. You will need to sit comfortably on a chair and have with you a pad of paper and a pen. Imagine an "X" mark on the floor to your right that represents the change that you want to make, and an "X" to your left side. The "X" mark on the left side represents the negative reasons that you have to make the change in your life and the "X" on the right side represents positive ones.

On the paper write the reasons you want to make the change. For example, let's say that the decision you want to make is about a change in career. Write on the paper the thoughts that have crossed your mind. Use one piece of paper per thought about the issue. (It is important to follow these steps carefully.) Now, decide if the thought you've written is negative or positive and put the paper to your left or right side. Use the guide on page 9 to help you determine whether your thoughts are positive or negative.

As you can see, on the column for thoughts I have underlined the negative comments. On the fourth example the word but is underlined because the "buts" are so big in our lives. You truly have to listen closely when you speak. Until you change your internal dialogue and are able to do this spontaneously, it is best to do this exercise by writing it on pieces of paper. Doing this will change the thinking positive and acting negative attitude that most people have without realizing why their lives are so difficult. Once you have identified your thought process about the issue, you can transform it and move all your thoughts to the positive side.

When you finish transforming your thought process, written now with only positive reasons, you will feel much more enthusiastic and energized to move forward and take the necessary steps to become or do. Every step of the way becomes more pleasurable because you have created a happy and positive future for yourself. What seemed to be big obstacles in the road are now the building stones and success is within reach! Congratulations! You truly do have the inner power to transform your life.

I have created a transformational workbook for my clients that enter the Honor Your Inner Treasures™ Program and as we go through the process they do simple, fun and motivating change processes. When they finish, only then the realization comes regarding how powerful it is to invest time into loving ourselves.

BELIEFS

All people have beliefs that help structure their lives. We know with great certainty that whatever we believe is true, and one of these beliefs is self-worth. People even determine their income based on their belief of self-worth. Your resume indicates exactly how much money you will make in the next year. When you review it and no changes have been made, you are hoping that inflation or the economy of the company you work for will determine the increase in the salary that you will be earning. Have you ever stopped to think about it? You are giving your power to another person to determine your growth, not only in your economy, but also your personal potential to do more, to become who you want to be.

I have worked with clients who are business owners feeling stressed out because of low funds, poor self-esteem and a lack of confidence. These issues not only impact their personal lives but also how their business grows. Those negative beliefs, ideas and limitations also have an impact on their earnings and the status of their finances, and all the people working for their company.

I remember working with Priti, a 43-year-old married woman. She emigrated to Canada from India, where she had received her degree as a software engineer. Once in Canada, Priti was able to obtain a position where she could use some of her education and experience. The reason I say 'some' of her education and experience is because when she came to see me for the first time she said that she was starting to feel bored with her job and not living up to her full potential. Priti felt that there were problems in the company that took too long to solve and required great work to make operations run more efficiently. Doing things the way the company had done for years was causing the same problems over and over again. She wanted to make a change and had a vision to do so.

However, Priti was quiet and didn't like to be the center of attention, so she kept to herself, trying to fit into the company's mold. Eventually, the conflict between shyness and wanting to change operations caused her a great deal of stress. She could not feel confident putting forth her suggestions. And although there was nothing I could do to help her with her software issues, I was able to help her build her confidence to act, speak, think and move forward. With those new positive traits, she was able to increase her self-esteem and recognize her own value.

Being foreign and fearing she might appear ignorant to others was one of Priti's greatest stumbling blocks. To offset this, I offered a metaphor. I asked her to consider the plastic casing that envelops the computer containing the software she created. Is that foreign? Obviously, the answer is no. The casing is just another part of the whole computer just as she, too, is part of the whole.

In creation nothing is foreign. We are all co-creating contributing our energy into the amazing universe we all live in. This is why it is so important that you truly live your lives from your inner treasures because underneath your fears and doubts you are pure potential, everyone has amazing positive energy to add to the whole.

We also worked on Priti's self-esteem and confidence by training her subconscious mind to act, feel and think the way the leader she desired to be would. The leader she wanted to be was one who confidently and clearly communicated her views, ideas and solutions with the tone of a manager. In just a few weeks Priti noticed she was expressing her ideas, asking questions and sharing her knowledge and experience without feeling timid. Most importantly, she noticed that her peers welcomed her ideas.

Eventually, Priti realized this company didn't have potential to grow and she was putting all of her potential in a box too small for her. She knew she was ready to move on with confidence.

That spark of inner realization of your personal self, and of how truly valuable your contribution is to everything you do, changes everything. You become confident to plan and live your life making decisions that feel right, and feel an inner peace because you gained control. Now, you have the power to do the things that are truly important to you. Once you learn to expand your consciousness beyond your fear, the limitation you had becomes limit-less.

In my upcoming book, *Limitless Beliefs - 7 Steps to Transcend into a Joyful and Abundant You*, you will find the how-to for this process. To purchase, learn more about the book, www.limitlessbeliefs.com or www.celinatioauthor.com.

YOUR LIFE IS YOUR DECISION AND YOUR CREATION

"Create your life experiences in such a way that the day you look back all you see is a magical garden of your own design that you can be proud of having imagined,

lived, grown and created." – Celina Tio

"Really? Are you sure? Because I was told…" These are all comments based on a lack of confidence. This does not have to be you! You are able to declare your independence, power and freedom! To embrace the true and pure intention of creation!

I'll share with you the experience of Laura, a beautiful and intelligent woman who came to my office for help. As she introduced herself and explained the reason why she had made the appointment, I was amazed. At 32 years old, she was a successful fashion designer. Her passion, however, was singing and songwriting. What an amazing girl, and what a disparity in her professional career compared to her dreams.

Her narrative was sad due to many of her life's circumstances and events. Her self-esteem and confidence was at an all-time low after ending a relationship that was going nowhere. Now, she hoped to let go of all her little self. Laura wanted to have more confidence to make decisions and communicate her ideas and feelings, and she wanted to feel good about herself. Simply put, she wanted to live happily.

I could have told her how beautiful, amazing and intelligent I thought she was. I could have pointed out all the wonderful opportunities she could have in life or how much I admired her. But she wasn't there for me to tell her what most any friend would. She needed to know from her own heart, discovering and loving herself so that she could go through her life's journey knowing her essence.

At the end of her journey I asked Laura to write what she decided was most valuable about herself. She took a few days and sent me an e-mail describing her value as she perceived it. Imagine the courage it took to be so vulnerable. Without relying on anyone else's opinions, she confessed her own beauty, strength, warmth and intelligence. She had honored her inner treasures.

I have asked her permission to share this with you because I want you to know that it is also possible for you. She kindly and happily agreed because she felt she could help other people. Maybe that person today is you or someone you love.

"I value myself because I am a strong person who perseveres through hardship, and I have faith I will get through it. I value myself because I am loving and kind-hearted person. I value myself because I take care of those in need and treat them just as I would treat myself. I value myself because I am a hard worker and very motivated. I value myself because I am a good woman. I value myself because I have self-respect and integrity, and will not allow anyone to take that away. I value myself because I am humble in life. I value myself because I am a good sister, friend, daughter, and lover because I care for people's feelings. I value myself because of my relationship with God and how I want to continue to help myself be better. I value myself because I am a loving woman who shares love with everyone. I value myself because I can make people laugh and really bring out the best in them; this shows me how amazing I am. I value myself because even if I am scared or fearful I have courage to face those fears. I value myself because of my ability to forgive and make amends even when people have truly hurt me. I value my positive thinking and my ability to turn what can be a bad situation into a great one. I value myself because I am able to express my feelings and my emotions now in a calm and mature way. I value myself because any goal I set for myself I achieve, because I am willing to work hard. I value myself because I always keep on smiling even when the going gets tough. I value myself because I am beautiful, strong, smart, mature, funny, loving, and kind person."

\- Laura, Toronto, Canada
Fashion Designer/ Singer and Songwriter, naturally from the heart.

APPRECIATION

If life were a coin, would you say it is less valuable when you are looking on the head side just because the imprinted value is on the other side and you can't see it?

The value of everything is found through deep appreciation. Lots of people walk through life with the expectation of being accepted and liked by others, but they suffer a great deal when the world around them doesn't show them what they expect. Start increasing your self-value by appreciating your life as it is in this moment. Even if your world looks or feels different than you'd like, there is value to be found. You can increase that value by describing it and saying thank you. At first, it might take some creativity if you have been depreciating things most of your life.

Let's think of something you do every day, like eating. All of us eat when we are hungry, but some also eat when anxious, nervous or depressed. There is even a name for this: comfort food. Comfort food is supposed to make you feel better when you eat it; however, nobody has ever said, "I was feeling sad and I ate a whole bowl of ice cream and now everything is fine! All of a sudden I feel loved and my finances have improved drastically with every spoonful of food I ate!" This would simply not be true.

On the other hand, when you eat because you feel hungry your body and mind feel better because they receive the nourishment needed. If you offer and share your meal and spend time in the company of family or friends, your soul is nourished as well. In preparing your meal, be grateful that you have the ingredients on hand needed to prepare the meal that will nourish every cell in your body. Imagine all the minerals, vitamins, proteins, carbohydrates and fibers that are present in what you are about to consume, and how you are benefiting from them. Thank the supermarket for having them available for you, and the people who've dedicated their life into growing them. Even thank the work you do that earns you the funds to buy your food. It's crucial to become aware of the dimension of what you are about to eat.

- Be grateful to the soil that has the perfect nutrients to grow your food.

- Be grateful to the sun and the water for adding their energy.

- Be grateful to the universe for having created a planet that contains everything you need.

- Be grateful for the beauty of the colors, textures and aromas of the vegetables, herbs or fruits, or a cup of coffee.

- Be grateful to the person who will share this meal with you.

- Be grateful that you can share your moment with that person and have each other's company.

- Be grateful that you have the ability to offer and share your meal.

- Be grateful that life is allowing this moment to sit, rest, replenish, keep each other's company and share whatever it is that needs to be shared at the moment.

By now, appreciation has started to flow from the heart and you will know if what you are about to eat is healthy for you. If you have to thank the chemicals named on the package that are so difficult to pronounce instead of the natural sweet aroma of a natural ripe tomato, you will know not to eat it. Your body will show you resistance. When appreciation flows from the heart, you will feel true comfort even when you drink plain water. Do it at your next meal. Do the same with your home, your family, your pet and your neighbor.

Practicing heartfelt appreciation will change your perspective on life.

SELF-REALIZATION

"You have the power of pure energy within you to be, to do, to have, to accomplish, to become your dream." – Celina Tio

When you truly know your essence, everything changes easily. Your relationships are healthier by helping you grow with people who share your life's path. Life becomes pleasurable and enjoyable, and conflict and stress no longer emanate from you. You understand that ego makes peoples lives sad and full of problems, and that it drives competition, fear, war and destruction.

Knowing your essence also means the things that you're doing now are in line with what makes you feel happy. It's easy to identify if you're off balance because life no longer feels whole. You become aware of your energy and how it affects everything around you. You have a fresh understanding that you are part of creation, co-creating with all that makes us one.

You become more independent when you know your essence, investing into your wellbeing and happiness instead of things that have no value to your personal self. Rich and wealthy has a whole different meaning now. No more spending to do things or obtain things just because you feel bored or empty. You'll no longer feel the need to shop in an attempt to feel happy or, even worse, to look happy. You become independent and know that you are the only one responsible for how you are living your life, with no one else to blame. Vacationing to escape from reality is a thing of the past. Instead, you'll have the freedom to choose a destination that will give you enjoyment in everything from the planning to the adventure to the return.

At this point, inner peace has become real in your life and you'll have the self-realization that you truly are the creator of every moment in your life. Your future is right this moment, so make it amazing and wonderful. Move from the comfort spot of sameness, obedience and unhappiness. Walking on your self-pity will take you only to more of the same. It is time to tell yourself that you deserve to experience life, and to savor and indulge in the sweetness and pure love of creation. You deserve to feel free of unnecessary pain, have inner peace and feel truly loved.

Of course we all have sad moments in our lives. It is normal to experience loss and birth, laughter with tears of joy and also tears of sadness, and expansion and contraction. It is the Yin and Yang of life. What's important is what you do with it.

Your inner being has been waiting for you to listen truthfully to the pureness within. You are powerful beyond your comprehension, and have more than strength. You have the power of pure energy within you to be, to do, to have, to accomplish, and to become your dream. When I realized how powerful I was created to be, I stopped feeling small. I rid myself of unnecessary fears, choosing instead to be one with the moment. I learned to breathe moments out of love, peace and joy, and to share it with you and everyone around me. Let me help you heal. Allow me to guide you into that place of discovering and once and for all Honor Your Inner Treasures. Your life will be transformed.

www.honoryourinnertreasures.com

www.limitlessbeliefs.com

www.celinatioauthor.com

You are Born to Have Joy

LYKKE STJERNSWÄRD

Many of you dream to actualize your potential, but you do not always know how to do so. I say, free yourself from your fears, take personal responsibility, be open to individual transformation, choose an active existence and contribute to an evolving society. Stand up and stand tall to make those choices and decisions that empower you and support positive change that resonates throughout communities and across time throughout generations. Connect and create the opportunity to make a difference, and know the value you are adding to the world.

I encourage you to connect to the present moment because joy is right in front of us for the taking. When we are mindful, we understand that the only life we have is the one we are living in now, and it is in the moment, the now, that we can shape our future. Tremendous power arises from recognizing this simple truth – that you're born to have joy in your life and in your work, and that you are your own key to living with passion and to enjoying every day as a gift. You come naked to the world. It is within you to build what you want in life.

My book *Born to Have Joy: Steps to Living the Life of a Gypset* shows you how you can step out of the conventional, to create an unconventional positive, joy-filled life that takes you out from the ocean of sameness and to make you a celebrity in your own life.

A cross of two words, Gypsy and Jet Set and coined by Julia Chaplin, author of Gypset Travel, it refers to a semi-nomadic bohemian lifestyle, a spirit of pure freedom "which fuses the ease and carefree lifestyle of a gypsy with the sophistication of the jet set. Gypsetters are artists, surfers, designers and bon vivants who live and work around the globe, from Jose Ignacio, Uruguay and Ibiza, Spain to Montauk, New York," describes Chaplin in her book. If you are a Gypsetter, you will be living an entrepreneurial life, inspiring others to think different inside the box, enjoying a nonconformist lifestyle and setting up your own guidelines for innovative businesses.

A Gypset life is based on a philosophy that a good life is lived at any moment and anywhere and that joy is found not in collecting things, but in experiences – reading a book at sunset on a deserted beach, sharing a home-cooked meal on a rooftop under candlelight in Goa or blending into the local culture, speaking the local language and engaging in community projects. Travelling off the beaten track and immersing in local cultures is part and parcel of the

Gypset style. So is standing out, trusting that your vision is important to the world and that you have the creative power and influence to inspire joy in your life and in the life of your community.

There are many opportunities for joy, and the first step is to recognize that the only life you have is the one you have now. You can absolutely shape or reshape your future, but you do so, not from fear or overplanning, from anxiety or overdoing, it is in the present moment where you love the life that you live that you are your most powerful.

As a photographer, I focus on the light of my client's inner being: his or her visible heart. I've found that the moment they are in touch with their inner glow, their path ahead is illuminated. As an entrepreneur and a founding creator of 8value.com, along with my fellow design partners, we work with change-makers, creating their brands by expressing their values visually. What that means is that we help you to know your value and to create your own personal brand that integrates your values, which are fundamental to differentiating yourself from others, adding vitality to your business, creating success, and bringing joy to your clients.

As part of our service, we give visual form to these values and help you design promotional items such as creating holistic satin ribbon or silicone bracelets with inspiring sayings such as *"The cure for fear is love"* or *"To be is to live here and now."* Think of them as little vessels or holders of your values to widen your influence by spreading joy.

By raising the visibility of your values, by helping your build relationships of trust and anticipating innovative solutions, we empower you to be a change-maker that stands for vision, innovation and sharing. In 8value.com, we encourage you to thrive on your own talent, invest your own time and energy where you love to make a difference, find hideouts and people with the perfect vibe that resonate and align with your desires, values, thoughts and actions. As a change-maker with game-changing solutions, you can create in and invest in something new birthed from your innovative vision that contributes to gross national happiness, not just gross national product.

LIVING AS A LEADER IN A SPIRIT OF FREEDOM

I've created a simple map for you to live the life of goodwill in *"Born to have Joy"* with simple-to-follow steps plus supportive guidance on which is the related chakra to work on for each move forward. By fine-tuning the energy centers and ensuring that body, mind and spirit are in perfect balance, you optimize your health, which is integral to living this life of freedom. I show you exciting destinations, both within and without, where you can thrive and be at your most creative, to be the artist of your own life. Since this is a journey of transformation and inspiration, akin to shedding old skin, I also recommend the appropriate affirmation engraved on a lucky charm bracelet from my collection at femininsacre.net to help connect your heart to your desire and to amp up your positive vibes to attract what you desire.

Here is a summary of the 8 steps:
1. Trust, respect and create a new you
2. Spot the opportunities for Joy
3. Foster joy and vitality by doing and loving what pleases you
4. Trust that you can always access infinite resources within you
5. Embrace quality time
6. Indulge in vital moments
7. Be creative and laugh a lot
8. Invite joy into your secret garden

1. Trust, Respect and Create a New You

This is a process of transformation to create visibility for yourself by finding your inner glow to light your path ahead. Decide what you want to do, knowing that your life has a finite end, and ensure you keep a healthy balance between mind, body and spirit. Empower yourself by respecting your need for space and do not be afraid to say no. Be your own genuine self to become the celebrity in your own life, create a life game plan and know that you are the key to your own success.

2. Spot Opportunities for Joy

Life is to be lived and engaged with in the present. You find joy in small things that matter such as a comforting hug or a friendly smile. You discover joy in building connections of the heart, working with others whom you trust and with whom you are in perfect harmony to create a common purpose to invest in something new for a great return on fun. Find something that contributes to happiness as well as to traditional economic measures of economic value.

On my own personal path, every day I choose three reasons for which to be grateful, to feel joy here and now, to love in the present and to live for the future.

3. Foster Joy and Vitality by Doing and Loving What Pleases You

Vitality is sourced in trust, and the key to building trust, the lack of which creates sadness, is transparency. Trust is fostered by loving in the present, each day experiencing the power of awareness of the moment. Invite a bright future into your life, one where you put in time and energy into something or somewhere you love making a difference. As a change maker, create an action plan, a life's game plan that builds on all these elements, that enhances joy and promotes vitality. Be celebratory, grab the momentum of the moment, bring colors into your life because if you love the life you live, you will live a life of love.

4. Trust that You Can Always Access Your Infinite Resources

In your inner world, your emotions pose challenges, but you can make friends of your emotions by giving each of them a name. On my journey, there is no room for envy, but if an emotion like jealousy springs up, I regard it as a friend bearing a message, a warning that I should either adapt to the situation or let go of whatever it is I'm hanging onto too tightly. Whether you rely on therapy or creative pursuits such as writing to become acquainted with your emotions, trust in your intuition as your best guide. It is your personal radar, and it will never mislead you. By trusting my intuition to tell stories around the world through photography, I now have a chance to display and share what I see through the lens with love and compassion. My jewelry brand, Féminin Sacré™, has given me a voice and connects me with my sisters in humanity.

Your life is yours to create, so create new opportunities and new challenges for yourself. I choose sport as the arena in which I find new ways to stretch myself, such as paragliding in Verbier or heli-skilling on untracked, pristine trails over steep cliffs in Le Petit Combin in the Swiss Alps. We all have it within us to be daredevils.

5. Embrace Quality Time

No matter where your Gypset life leads you, everyday remind yourself that positive thinking is the most untapped natural resource in the world, and it doesn't run out on you! Surround yourself with loving, positive vibes that nurture and foster creativity.

Invite love into your life, starting with your body, which is your temple. Every day open to daily awareness by performing a salutation to the sun and including the ones you love and yourself in daily prayers. Such simple but heartfelt steps immersed in gratitude are easily introduced into your own life to support you, to maximize your health, to tap fully into your potential. Remember, the most thrilling way to enjoy life is to be the best part of yourself.

6. Indulge in Vital Moments

Schedule time for yourself, but also allocate time to at least three to five essential projects in your life. Like the legs of a chair, even if one falls off, the chair is still usable on three legs. If one of your projects fail to take off, you have at least 2 to 3 others working for you.

In other moments, cultivate a winning attitude. My own winning attitude is rooted in a belief in an intelligent design that is mightier than me. Being told "God loves me" and "I will pray for your both" are some of the most impactful words I have ever heard. What is your winning attitude? Find clues by taking responsibility for your thoughts and actions, build positive dialogue and ensure that your actions have a beautiful quality. Be mindful with your actions, be open, cool, sophisticated and purposeful.

7. Be Creative and Laugh a Lot

'Creativity is intelligence having fun' - Albert Einstein

In Toltec wisdom, life is considered as art. You are the artist and your life, every aspect of it, every act, every day, every moment, is an expression of yourself as an artist. If your life is a blank canvas, what will you paint on it?

Where will you live? Find the cities and countries that fuel your creativity, spur your mobility and celebrate your freedom.

I suggest to you as a guide the books of Bobo Karlsson, a Swedish author now resident in Rio de Janeiro, who has been dubbed "Sweden's best urbanista". In his two books, *Urban Safari* and *Urban Safari 2*, he writes about his favorite cities and describes the souls and energies of cities such as Mexico City, whose mayor won the World Mayor Prize in 2010 for radically reducing pollution and improving the environment, and Berlin, whose mayor, Klaus Wowereit attracted the young to his city by creating the mantra "Penniless and Sexy". Cities have energies. Find the one that activates the creativity in your DNA.

8. Invite Joy into Your Own Secret Garden

Your secret garden is the little place in your heart where you spend time in to regain your equilibrium. Sometimes, you need a little help from outside to help you connect with your own secret garden. In Geneva, I use a unique transformational massage, Tulayoga, at Insens to heal myself with the help of my body.

You grow your secret garden by living with passion. Every day, laugh and dance, invite people into your life by hosting events that celebrate living. Join the party by linking the world for a worthy cause, meet new people and create new opportunities for yourself. In the words of Doña Esra, Toltec Wisdom teacher, "You have the right to be happy."

I've shared with you a little of the know-how so you can live a freedom and passion-fuelled life, one in which you are the star of your own show. I hope I've raised the bar for excitement to show that you can live free and create new change-making empowering opportunities while feeling fully confident you have access to unlimited resources to attract what you desire into your life. By shedding the stories that put you down, by filling the space with a winning attitude, by encouraging you to take responsibility for your thoughts and action, by linking to others with positive vibes, I assure you life as a Gypset is yours for the taking.

A lucky dreamer, explorer, photographer, entrepreneur and author, Lykke Stjernswärd has certainly lived up to her name, which means 'Happy Star Sword' in Swedish. A graduate of the Art Center College of Design in Switzerland and the University of Geneva she holds a B.A. in Communication Design and another in entrepreneurship and business development. With an international portfolio of photography, Lykke has worked on assignments for *Vogue* Nippon and her portraits have been published in *The New York Times* and *The Herald Tribune*. Her work is seen across the globe in London, Budapest, Hong Kong, Stockholm, Geneva and Riga, as well as on www.lykke.ch. Lykke's offers holistic fashion jewelry, bracelets and charms at www.femininsacre.net. She is also the founder of www.8value.com, a company that serves to brand visionary and innovative change-makers.

To discover how you can love success in your life and believe it is transferable, please email Lykke at femininsacre@me.com

Go Ahead, Give Yourself Permission to Dream Big

BRIARLEY NICHOLSON

I saw my home go up in flames on Christmas Day, when I was barely seven. Our farm was invaded during the civil war in Zimbabwe (then Rhodesia), petrol poured over and around the house, a struck match thrown in. We escaped death because, fortunately, we were in the city of Harare with our grandmother on Christmas Eve, when the invasion occurred.

I escaped an attempted rape at school, when I was 11.

I grew up in a country where, at its worst, hyperinflation was officially 13.2 billion % per month. This meant that money had to be spent the moment it was earned because, come tomorrow, it wouldn't be worth the paper it was printed on. The good part was I became a trillionaire very quickly, and I still hold a $100,000,000,000,000 note (and 13 zero's have been removed!)

However, here I am. I wasn't born with a silver spoon in my mouth. Despite a currency whose value slipped like sand through the fingertips, and on occasion not having two cents to rub together, I've done the things I've set out to do, overcome the challenges, and become the person I sought to be. I love what I do, helping people transform to greater success, achieve financial freedom and live life with passion on their own terms.

I'm not anyone especially gifted. I wasn't an A student nor did I seek academic honours. I did, however, desire to travel and, by going for my dreams, I transitioned through South Africa as the first step, and then moved to London. I worked hard, saved, kept out of debt and travelled around the world, realizing my passion for global adventures.

I discovered that going for my dreams was easier than I ever thought possible, and it was a whole lot of fun.

I've made big leaps in personal transformation by studying first-hand with some of the world's greatest coaches including Tony Robbins, Robert Kiyosaki, Matt Morris, Marc Accetta, Johnny Wimbrey, Scott Harris, T. Harv Eker, Les Brown, Raymond Aaron, to name a few.

Along the way, I created a simple-to-follow system for financial empowerment that kept yielding consistent and repeatable successes. By adhering to tried and true strategies, I made huge quantum leaps in my life. My life is richer and fuller because I was willing to reach out for what life had to offer and take a chance.

Pretty good for a young farm girl from a small mining town, Bindura, in Zimbabwe.

Each of us has untold potential within us, and it's there for the taking, no matter the cards we've been dealt.

Do any of these sound familiar?

Weighed down by too much debt?

Trapped in an undesirable job?

Can't stop the spending habit?

Working too hard for too little?

Held back by fear and insecurities?

Feeling something's missing?

Finding instant gratification doesn't work?

Afraid of the future?

Feeling you're owed it, why should you work for it?

Never got time?

Do you want the next chapters of your life to be more of the same or do you want to live the life you've always dreamt of? If you say "yes" to a dream life with more ease, more fun, more success, read on.

TIME TESTED, EASY, MANAGEABLE PRINCIPLES

I'm going to share some of my success principles with you to create the financial freedom and independence you deserve. These are the same strategies that I use in my coaching consultations, my online seminars and my workshops.

1. Now is All You Have, Don't Waste it

The time that you have is your most precious commodity. Once it's come and gone, it stays gone. You can't rewind that clock nor reclaim the days, months and years you've lost. You can lose money and make more, but you can NEVER make more time.

What this means is that you act now. You take action now; even if they are small steps, you take them consistently, at full tilt.

There's no perfect moment when everything falls into place.

Maybe you are dithering and spinning "what ifs" in your head because you are afraid of making mistakes.

It's quite simple, really. If you do nothing while waiting for the perfect moment, nothing is what you get back. There is no perfect moment. Life is life.

2. Give Yourself Permission to Dream Big

Dream big, and then dream even bigger. It's your life, if you don't dare to dream the things you want, who's going to do it for you? Your family, your friends, your partner? No, they've their own lives to lead.

Maybe right now you're saying, "Briarley, that's just silly daydreaming. I dream of becoming a millionaire, but look at where I am. No way am I becoming a millionaire unless I buy a winning ticket."

Let me tell you otherwise.

Matt Morris, celebrated author and one of my mentors, was at 21 years homeless, $30,000 in the red, and lived out of the back of his car. By the time he turned 24, he was earning six-figures, and by 29 he had made his millions.

He gave himself permission to dream of being a millionaire. Starved and hungry in the back of his car, wishing for millions in his bank account was not very sensible or doable, was it? But he didn't doubt himself. Instead, he went after his dream, without looking back.

Don't edit yourself; instead raise the bar on your dreams.

Remember nothing happens without you first thinking or dreaming about it.

"If you can imagine it, you can achieve it. If you can dream it, you can become it"

"Winners Never Quit and Quitters Never Win"

These are my favorite quotes on success, and ones that I live by. You never give up on your dream. It may take longer than you expected, there may be a few more bumps on the road, but it is always possible. A great book that illustrates this most is "The Impossible Just Takes a Little Longer" by Art Berg. I always dreamed of having children and a family; life turned out differently, probably because of my independence, and when I started trying for kids I could not conceive. I was so determined at never quitting that, despite doctors telling me I had no eggs left and would have to get an egg donor, my mindset was right and I conceived naturally. Today I have the most amazing son, Ricky. DREAM and NEVER QUIT!!!

3. Fear is Just a Four-Letter Word

There is a space for such four letter words – the junk pile. Fear becomes bigger than it really is when we feed it, and it grows fat on our anxieties and concerns.

Some of you may fear failure. You worry that you'll become the laughing stock of your circle and lose any esteem in the eyes of others. You must have a strong reason WHY you want to achieve, to ignore the bystanders (because that is what they are).

But look at the success stories of today, pick any models of success, read up on their life stories and you'll see that what differentiated them was that they didn't let their fears hold them back. They stared fear in the face and, guess who flinched first? Not them. 99% of what one worries about never actually happens anyway.

Even if they made mistakes, and big ones too, these successful men and women took notes from their experiences and applied those lessons to becoming even more successful in the future.

When we see fear for really what it is – just a four letter word – we can hurdle over it and run forward with ease towards what we want.

4. Keep Your Eye on the Prize

I'm not going to lie and tell you it's easy. You may have to work harder than you've ever had to.

I held two jobs in South Africa for eighteen months to earn enough to buy my first airline ticket to London. Once there, I shared a house with 13 others, held three jobs -- a full-time secretarial job, weekend days as a sales representative, and weekend nights serving behind a bar. I worked hard, went without and made sacrifices.

By regularly depositing my salary into a savings account and living off my weekend earnings, I realized my dream of visiting exotic countries and immersing myself in colorful cultures.

Did I find it hard going? Sometimes, but I kept my eye on the prize – being a global traveler – and I kept going and had a blast doing so.

Later, trying to fall pregnant, I was faced with turbulent emotions, hormone imbalances, drugs and financial challenges. I observed unwanted pregnancies in other people, noticed neglected children, encountered the fear of never having a child, and the list goes on. It was not easy at all; however, I had my eye on the prize and only the prize. There was no room for doubt. I won!

That's because I realized that everything I did got me closer to my dreams.

5. MAP – A small word that packs a mighty punch

MAP stands for two things.

Firstly, it stands for map, the guidance system that you need to get you from here to there.

If you were driving a car, you'll turn on your GPS system, figure how long it will take, get fuel to make sure you are not stranded, and turn on the music (in my case, it is Personal Development). If it's a long journey, you may look for place to refuel and renew. You'll find the data you need to guide you along the pathway with a map.

MAP also stands for Massive Action Plan, and it starts with being very clear with your goals. By knowing what you want to achieve and why, you identify the true purpose behind a goal.

Once you understand true purpose, you'll be able to connect the dots between desire, action and results.

You'll be able to monitor whether you are taking the right steps that are producing the right outcomes, or whether you are being side-tracked by detours or non-essential action.

You get three powerful benefits out of a MAP.

I. It Provides Clarity

Many people quit because they lose their sense of direction. They get bored. And they end up where they don't want to be.

A MAP allows you to correct course. If you feel you're pursuing the wrong goal, you know to go back to basics.

Understand the purpose why you are reaching for a specific goal. As you probe beneath the surface, you may realize you have set this goal because it's expected of you. Not because you really want it for yourself.

Time to reset and get back on track.

II. It Strengthens Commitment

You get to pat yourself on the back and celebrate when you get results that you desire. Knowing that you're doing absolutely the right things towards your goals is a pretty big motivator. It lifts you up and fills you with positive, boundless energy. When you're so filled with such excitement and energy, you're unstoppable.

That's massive action.

III. It Empowers

MAP is result-orientated. By breaking what you need to do into small, specific steps, you kick-start yourself into making moves and, before you know it, you're that much closer to your goals because of the momentum you've created.

More importantly, you're self-directing the action towards your goals to realize your desires.

You're taking back control, rather than being controlled by external circumstances. That's real power.

These are some of the dynamic strategies available to you to turn your life around, wire into the potential that lies within and create greater fulfillment.

HERE'S EVEN MORE GOOD NEWS

An exciting journey lies ahead of you, to move from financial distress to financial empowerment, from a ho-hum life to a life of greatness. Here are a few more lessons I learned along the way, on my own path to discovery.

• Passion turns hard work into fun

All of us have experienced this. We don't notice time passing, we are not bothered by distractions and we even forget when we are hungry when we are fully engaged in something that fires up our passion.

Passion taps into your own personal power and strengths, some of which may be hidden. It is your fuel when the going gets bumpy and it is your best weapon to make your dreams come true.

Look within to find out what fires you up.

• Commit, follow through, be accountable

Commitment follows from purpose. It's easy to stay gung-ho when the going is easy but what happens when it becomes challenging?

Stay focused. Remind yourself it is your life, remember your purpose, keep walking forward, remain curious. Life rewards you greatly when you dare. Think abundance not scarcity.

Turn up when you say you will, deliver what you promise to do, and be responsible for your successes and your mistakes.

By always following through and staying accountable, you are shaping within yourself a priceless habit of consistency. When you do it often enough, like any habit, it becomes second nature and it stays with you for life.

• You don't have to walk alone

A journey of a thousand steps may seem like a very lonely path. Here's the good news. You don't have to do it alone.

There are workshops, mastery seminars, masterminded groups, online forums, like-minded travelers, mentors, coaches. There are boundless resources and opportunities.

Reaching out for your dreams sounds like a big lofty idea. However, I support you with easy, practical and manageable how-to-tips in my book, online courses and coaching consultations that can be applied immediately. You get simple, solid steps for how to take action now; not next week or next month, but right now.

They are time-tested how-to tips and proven strategies. As you achieve successes in small steps, you can add more and more as you feel comfortable to build up momentum towards financial empowerment, freedom and a purposeful, fulfilling life.

The next step is yours to take.

A successful life and financial transformational coach, Briarley Nicholson is an entrepreneur and has her own successful businesses in financial advisory, money management, management accounting, network marketing, coaching and property investing, and loves to travel and meet people. Briarley is passionate about using her professional training and life experiences to make a difference in people's lives. She helps her clients develop breakthrough strategies to achieve financial freedom and design a life of their dreams.

Email: briarleynicholson@gmail.com
Website: www.WhySettleForGoodWhenGreatAwaitsYou.com
Tel: +1 727 214 5977

Awakening Your Healer Within

The Miracle of You!

PHILIP YOUNG

In this book you will glean information from "authorities" who offer mind-expanding ideas and concepts that will benefit your entire life and wellbeing. After countless hours of extensive study, thousands of client sessions, and twenty-five years experience, I am excited to be an authority. In my case, the particular subject of expertise is energetic healing and, like the other authorities in this book, I am pleased to share some of this information and knowledge with you. When learned and understood correctly, energetic healing has the ability to uplift, enlighten, and heal either you or a loved one.

To begin, we must define energetic healing. This is a metaphysical healing that takes place beyond the limits and assumptions of physical science known today. In reading this, you will learn how your inner, non-physical energy affects your health and wellbeing, and how this non-physical energy can be harnessed to assist you, sometimes in miraculous ways.

Today, most people see good health as something that is outside of their control, something that they have to fight to maintain. Health is also usually seen as that which is administered to them by outside medical experts and specialists, but there is another approach. What would it be like if, instead of seeking immediate traditional medical assistance, we embraced and recognized the body's own infinite wisdom? Could we then make changes from within? As people are able to open their minds to it, the answer to this question is most emphatically yes. All the wise and experienced physicians I've met with agree that, even with the scientific knowledge that has been gained over the years, we still know very, very little about the complexities of the human body. We are just beginning to scratch the surface of the miracle that we are.

The point of mentioning how little we know is to emphasize that there is another way of being, a way that truly 'does no harm' and is ultimately within your own control and power. If chosen, this is a path that leads to a radiant, healthier, and happier life that will help fill you with greater joy and wonder than ever before experienced.

Let's start with history. In ancient times it was understood that the natural state of human beings was one of vibrant health, and that this vibrant health came from the Self within. As science progressed, facts and data began to take precedence and this inherent knowledge was lost, buried, changed, or distorted. Now, millennia later, these truths are slowly being rediscovered.

I'd like to suggest that the secret of your entire health lies within you, and it is something that you can control with intention. It is something to be conscious of and to take responsibility for. This is a concept seldom taught or understood, which is especially regrettable because it takes so little commitment and discipline. In much the same way as other daily habits become routine, such as brushing your teeth, taking control of your health can be just that easy.

Many people regard themselves as victims or survivors of a disease (dis-ease), and this attitude has been encouraged in various ways in our society. It is a viewpoint that diminishes the Self and gives power to others. As you begin to consider yourself empowered as an active director of your own health, you engage your mind, spirit and body with intent, allowing miraculous changes to occur.

Every moment of every day, millions of cells are being created perfectly within your lungs, your organs, and your blood. All this takes place at the will of non-physical energy and is without any conscious effort on your part. It occurs simply by your inherent desire and intent. This is a monumental clue to the Truth and the beginning of realizing that you already are a miracle! This non-physical energy fills and actually enlivens your cells, tissues, and even your DNA. In fact, it permeates your entire being. Without being too esoteric, think of it as a 'Life Force', one that ultimately gives you Life and also determines your level of health and wellbeing. In circumstances when your health may not be currently optimal, this energy may have been compromised in some way. However, with help, application and some minimal training, it can be redirected to once again be a positive and beneficial resource for your body.

The dilemma that we have in our limited and often blinkered western way of looking at the world is that this non-physical energy has yet to be measured by material instruments. Society as a whole believes that, if something can't be measured, it cannot be. This line of reasoning actually mimics that of well-meaning priests from medieval times, who might have rigorously dismissed the concept of radio waves simply because they did not have the means to measure them at the time. That way of thinking is archaic. Non-physical energies can be perceived by those who are trained and considered to be attuned, open, and intuitively gifted. Moreover, the effects of these energies can be seen and experienced by all, whether or not we are aware of them.

For many years I have had the good fortune to help people experience healings that have been described as miraculous and even impossible. The people who have experienced healing have been able to reach a certain place within them of greater possibility. The process felt so natural, gentle, and effortless for them that they were often not even consciously aware of it taking place. In much the same way that you can use a magnifying glass to ignite kindling or paper, with my assistance people are able to reach a place of perfect health, a place Within that they ordinarily could not reach on their own.

So, how on earth do you reach the place Within that is already perfect? It is similar to tuning in to a radio station. In this case, however, you are tuning in to a subtle part of your Self. Continuing the radio metaphor, you may well experience some static, but if you persist you are able to tune in to that perfect part of you. As you invite the energy to come forth, hold a strong and consistent intent. Don't give up. When people struggle with this, occasionally they'll recall how they were when they were little children: carefree, happy, and hopefully in perfect health. A child's mind is filled with the exact joyfulness, openness and trust you are seeking. By holding onto these memories, the process may be easier.

To tune in to this station, it is also important to maintain a conscious feeling of gratitude for your perfect health in this very moment, regardless of present outward appearances. It's also important to suspend the activities of the intellect and ego and to control the mind chatter. You must move gently and in a state of deep relaxation through your feeling Self and through your loving Heart. By allowing yourself to maintain this thankfulness and gratitude for the miracle that you are, you can continue to fine tune this channel of perfection.

Because the process is unfamiliar, it can seem difficult at first. Most people find it far easier to begin with my help, and they always have beneficial results when they do. This occurs simply by my being fully Present with individuals in each visit with them. I speak with and listen to each person with patience and compassion. Using the vibration of my voice, and the heat and healing touch of my hands both on and around my clients' bodies, I'm able to help them find that place of perfection that's Within.

Over the years, I have found that there are always emotional hurts and concerns (real or imagined) that affect the wellbeing of the individual. Often, there are few if any people who have the time, patience, or compassion, and who are willing to listen to these concerns, much less respond in a supportive and loving way. Many doctors and specialists I meet sadly agree that they only have a few minutes to spend with each patient. Seldom do they learn much about the individual's hopes, past, fears, loves, concerns, personalities, relationships or families. So for them, if that were the case, it just wouldn't be possible to determine how non-physical energies may be of help to those in need.

When I meet clients in need of non-physical healing I allow the vibration of unconditional Love and highest intention to come forth. These energies can be felt as heat in my hands. Sometimes people actually think I have electric heating pads placed on their body. My own body becomes very warm, even hot, as these non-physical energies flow. It is a process of surrendering, of trusting without any ego whatsoever. Something much, much greater is present and in control. Usually this occurs for about an hour and then the energies stop, as the individual is complete. It is much the same way as we stop pouring water into a glass when it is full. No more can be added for the time being.

I feel most blessed to share these deep, sacred insights into the world of each individual. It allows for another aspect of their health, wellbeing and hope to blossom forth and then they feel better. True healing has to consider the totality of the person. It's a matter of body, mind, and spirit.

The following pages chronicle a few of the positive results I've obtained during my many years of practice. These anecdotal accounts demonstrate how real people have experienced wonderful results during healing sessions. Remember, if one man, woman, or child can do it, then so can another! Perhaps you are seeking a remedy at a time when other choices seem dim. If so, it could be that I might be able to help you or a loved one in some way. Whatever the reason, our Hearts and minds have crossed here for a sacred reason. I do hope that you enjoy the material on these pages and that you are inspired to implement the ideas for yourself, or perhaps to share them with others. Within the sanctity and authority of your own Self, take Heart, remain hopeful, and have faith that another way is surely at hand.

BREAST CANCER

"Your breasts are all clear."

Many years ago a dear and beloved friend called one day to say she had breast cancer. Little did I know then that her journey would help me embark on my own journey to becoming a healer.

Trish had been diagnosed with breast cancer and she was dreading the usual medical approach of "cut, poison, and burn" that still today seems to be the one size fits all medical standard. She had been endeavoring to learn as much as possible about her disease, including various alternative ways to treat her condition. She was fearful of chemotherapy's associated toxicity and the side effects that she knew would be so debilitating for her long-term health and wellness. She was open to another approach that was not harmful to her.

After many years of my own esoteric studies and interests, I was now faced with the stark reality of speaking my truth and endeavoring to do something for her or saying nothing while still trying to be supportive. Many of us have often found ourselves in similar situations. It's a matter of walking the talk vs. talking the talk.

I asked Trish if she was willing to try some healing after she had a lumpectomy. She answered yes and was, in fact, willing to try anything that might help. One day we sat down on her cottage lakefront and, to the bemusement of her husband and my wife, began to try a healing process I had read about. I felt certain and hopeful that I could really help her. That day, for about an hour we held the first of several such sessions, not really knowing what to expect, but highly desirous of a good outcome. Although these were just early steps at the time, nonetheless the good outcome arrived! Her breast cancer disappeared completely and to this day, over 20 years later, her breasts are cancer free!

LIFE SENTENCE

"We can't understand it. The tumors are gone."

Several months later I received a phone call from Jillian, a woman referred to me by Trish. Jillian had cancer throughout her body and had been diagnosed as only having a month or two to live. She was told to go home and get her affairs in order. We arranged to meet at her home and we spoke at length about what was going on in her life.

For the first five weeks we gently dealt with some personal issues that she had experienced. On each visit as I spoke with her I laid my hands upon her as she went into a deep guided relaxation. She returned to the hospital for follow up scans and tests, much to the amazement (and even anger, she said) of her medical doctors, as she had defied their diagnosis. Her tumors were either shrinking or had disappeared completely! Over the next several months she and I continued her healing sessions to the point where all tumors were completely gone.

I continued to see Jillian occasionally for over a two-year period. Years later, she eventually passed, but her life and vitality had been extended so much to the everlasting joy of her family, friends and loved ones.

COMA

"Your daughter is going to be in a permanent vegetative state. We are sorry, but there is no hope."

I happened to meet Rita by chance in an office where she was working. Rita told me her daughter Katrina had been struck by a car and had been thrown 70 feet. She had severe head trauma and had been in a coma for several weeks and, at this point, it was expected by the doctors that she would be in a permanent vegetative condition. There was nothing more they could do for her.

When I was a little boy I experienced head trauma and have always felt a deep sense of compassion and empathy for those who have head injuries. When Rita told me about Katrina, I knew that I had to see her. Out of the blue, I asked Rita if she would be open to that and she said yes.

The next day, walking down the corridors of the hospital, part of me was asking what in the world I was doing there. Part of me wanted to get out of there before I made a complete fool of myself. And yet, another part of me was serene, sure, and calm. I felt like something was guiding me.

Rita was already in Katrina's room and we exchanged a few words. The doctors would not know what I'd be doing, but a couple of the nurses had been informed so that we would not be disturbed quite so much. Seeing Katrina so unresponsive on her bed was quite unsettling. What was I going to say to her? How could this possibly work without a verbal exchange? Without any feedback? With no clues from the eyes? Then I felt a still, calm knowing within me that became my guide. I moved the bed out from the wall, leaned over, and put my hands gently on first Katrina's head, then arm, then hand. Her mom simply looked on, accepting. After about 45 minutes, the healing session seemed to be complete. I really didn't know what to expect. This was new territory for me.

A day later, Rita phoned me to tell me that Katrina had moved her thumb and that the doctors had said this was a reflex. I replied that this is exactly the type of reflex we wanted! A few days later I went back to the hospital and repeated the session, gently touching her arm, her heart, as well as her head. Rita phoned again with good news; this time that Katrina had moved her arm. When I checked my messages a couple of days later I heard one from Rita. Katrina had spoken! I was so overjoyed to hear that and tears ran down my face. It was Christmas Day – what a gift! I saw Katrina several more times and I'm so thrilled that she made a full and quite miraculous recovery.

BRAIN BLOOD VESSEL PROBLEMS (AVM)

"I could drop dead at any moment."

Len was recommended by a friend after he was told by the medical specialists that he had a very serious malformation in the thalamus of his brain. The condition is called an arterio-venous malformation or AVM. There was a weakening in the walls of the blood vessels feeding this very intricate and important region of the brain and he was enduring terrible headaches and some numbness in his extremities. His doctors explained that the medical treatment for such a condition was gamma knife brain surgery. If he survived at all, he could have many cognitive deficits. If he did nothing, he left himself at risk of the malformation erupting and of inevitable sudden death. The odds were against him.

I was his last resort and our first meeting was brief. He was short on time and clearly short on inclination to believe in non-physical healing. He told me that he also had tendonitis from playing golf and wondered if I could do something for that, too. Before long he was soon on the massage table in a deep sleep-like state.

I thought things had gone well and after an hour brought him back. He said he felt unusually relaxed, yet he also seemed to be skeptical as to what he had just experienced. Not surprising for such a practical left brain thinking, alpha male. Still, he was very gracious and we said our farewells.

Sometimes, clients will call me soon after our sessions to let me know their good news. I hadn't heard from Len for several weeks and I was beginning to think that perhaps things had not gone so well for him, but then my phone rang. "Hi Philip, it's Len. I've been meaning to call you. The numbness in my extremities that I'd had for two years was gone the very next day after our session. Also, my stress was relieved and my tendonitis is completely gone too! Most importantly, I had another follow up MRI and the malformation has apparently shrunken from the size of a quarter to the size of a dime. The need for surgery has been averted."

The doctors apparently were astonished by the outcome. They said it was impossible.

Over the following year or two, I heard from Len asking for my assistance on a few other matters, including on behalf of a friend who had hurt her right shoulder ten years previously and could find no relief. She called me the very next day after that session. "I don't know what you did, but all the pain is now gone."

EPILEPSY

"I could black out at any time. I'll never drive or ride again."

Christine and I first met in a metaphysical/spiritual bookstore. We had lots in common and we became great friends. She is also into fitness and health, with a thriving home-based business on a ranch north of Toronto. In addition to caring for her animals, one of her greatest passions is driving a Harley Davidson. Recently, she had been experiencing epileptic seizures and was on strong medications to try and keep the unpredictable seizures under control. The prospect of no longer being able to drive or ride was a huge issue for her.

She was open to having some healing sessions, so I went to her ranch. Christine had three sessions, all of which went well. She now has a full and normal life, teaches yoga, and continues to ride her beloved Harley!

BLOCKED SALIVA GLAND

"I can't eat or drink. The pain is unbearable."

It was a bleak Monday evening in early December. The door opened slowly to reveal a tall, elegant young woman. I smiled and introduced myself and her eyes searched my face for a fleeting second, looking for...what? Hope, perhaps? With a wince of pain, she smiled back slightly.

We sat in her living room and, after exchanging pleasantries, she described her medical condition. Judy could not eat and could barely drink. On a pain and discomfort scale she was at a 10 plus. Her sub-mandible saliva gland duct was blocked with a large stone nearly 6mm (¼ inch) in size. The gland had also become infected. A prominent ENT (ear, nose, and throat) specialist had tried unsuccessfully in a two-hour operation to surgically remove the stone. She sought second opinions and all the ENTs had told her that the only medical recourse was to have her entire saliva gland removed. As a doctor herself she knew that a life without a saliva gland would also be intolerable, not to mention that there could also be permanent nerve damage to her face. She simply had to explore another avenue of possibility, no matter how outlandish it might seem, and thus the call to me.

Judy and I continued to speak at length about what was and had been going on in her life, recently and in the more distant past. A discomfort in her neck and jaw had been part of her life for nine years that seemed to worsen during emotional upset and stress. To me there was an obvious connection, but often the person suffering does not see it.

Judy seemed to be open to the possibility of non-physical healing, so after about 45 minutes we began. With some soothing music playing, I spoke quietly to her as she lay on my healing table. Slowly, she drifted away into a sleep-like state while I placed my hands gently on, around, and above her jaw, mouth, and neck. We ended our session and agreed to meet again in two days. I provided her with some positive thoughts and affirmations to focus on before our next session, that would allow the conscious and unconscious mind to do their parts to support the process further.

When we met again Judy's spirits seemed brighter and she was excited to report that the pain she had been experiencing had reduced significantly from a 10 to a more tolerable 4. She was no longer taking any Percocet for the pain.. During our talk, Judy said that her concerns were now more with the blockage and swelling under her tongue and the discharge from the infection. She rated both of these as a 9 out of 10 on the misery scale.

I reminded Judy of the miraculous being she was already and emphasized that in each and every moment her physical body was performing millions and millions of complex functions without any conscious effort on her part. Her Essential Self was taking care of all these functions. I suggested that this is a part of her that is not generally known to the conscious mind, the ego, or intellect. On the table once again, she drifted off into a relaxed sleep-like state while the energies flowed gently and lovingly in and around her being. As we completed, we again agreed to meet in two days time.

On my third visit Judy told me that after our last meeting she had run to the bathroom and had to spit something out. Amazingly, she was also able to eat again! Judy was excited to tell me that the misery index for the swelling under her tongue and the infection was now only at a 2! The pain had gone. There was only a small bubble under her tongue and only a very slight discomfort on the left side of her neck.

I spoke to Judy a few weeks after that session. In the intervening time, she had had new x-rays that came back with the following reading: No calculi. The stone was completely gone!

ACID REFLUX

"For a long time I experienced the constant threat and misery of acid reflux disease."

Roy, a vital and distinguished gentleman, came to me at age 89. He had suffered with acid reflux for a long time, including a dreadful burning in his throat and stomach, and an appalling taste in his mouth. He had to be very careful about what and when he ate and would often be awakened during the night with great pain and discomfort. Roy's medical doctor had prescribed endless amounts of Gaviston pills for the symptoms but offered no actual remedy. The pills did little to relieve the unrelenting pain, discomfort, and burning sensation. The acidic, acrid taste in his mouth continued to be intolerable.

I asked Roy if he would like to have a healing session right there and then, where he stood chatting outside. He readily agreed (although he was concerned about what the neighbors might say!) I stood next to him and put my hand on his solar plexus and on his back. Right away, the energies began and I started to feel the familiar heat. We stood there for about 10 minutes and then we were complete.

The next day Roy reported that he had slept right through the entire night and that the burning feeling and taste was totally gone. In just one 10-minute session the condition completely disappeared!

It has been over a year now and Roy continues to be free of all the former acid reflux pain and discomfort and can pretty well eat whatever he likes.

"I'm overjoyed now to report that after just a few minutes with Philip, my discomfort has all but vanished!! It has truly been a life-changing experience for me. Philip is a miracle worker!"

SHOULDER AND NECK PAIN

"I don't know what you did, but my pain has been completely cured."

Whitney attended a special restorative yoga class of about a dozen people, where I was able to spend about six or seven minutes with each participant in a healing class setting. She reported that, in just those few minutes, I was able to completely heal her long-standing shoulder and neck problems.

KNEE PROBLEMS

"I can hardly walk, I can't skate. All my practice will be wasted."

Mary was a pre-teen figure skater. She had been unable to skate for some time due to a nasty fall. Her parents took her to physical therapists and specialists throughout the Toronto area with no success. Now, her father brought her to me, literally carrying her in. I spoke with Mary as she lay on a couch while her dad sat outside by the window enjoying the afternoon sun. As I spoke to her and put my hands on her knees and legs, she drifted off into a deep relaxation. After about an hour she was complete and said she felt as if she had been on a wonderful vacation and gave a vivid account of all kinds of beautiful colors while in this dream-like state. The next day, her parents were dumbfounded as they watched her perform skating jumps with ease.

Mary said, "After I saw you, I could walk again, and the very next day I was actually doing figure skating jumps for the first time in five months. I am not going to miss the nationals after all. Thank you so much!"

TEETH AND ROOT CANAL

"I have terrible tooth pain. Another root canal will cost me thousands!"

Over the years, Clare had had a number of painful and expensive root canals. Recently, the pain began again and her dentist recommended yet another. Clare had received a number of healing sessions from me for other health and wellness concerns and, when I asked her, said she was open to trying some healing on her jaw and teeth as well.

As she lay back deeply relaxed on her couch, I gently cradled her right jaw and touched her lower molars. After about an hour, we were complete and the next day, the pain had gone. Clare cancelled the root canal procedure with her dentist and is problem-free to this day. In just one session we eliminated the pain and we eliminated the issue.

FOOT PROBLEMS

"I'm afraid my life is over."

Hanna had severe foot problems and was not able to walk properly. Her job of 25 years required her to be mobile and on her feet all day so this issue was completely debilitating. When we met, I spoke to Hanna and explained to her about the strength and power of non-physical energies. I touched her arm and heart. After that the pain in Hanna's feet went away.

Hanna says, "I thought my life was over because I could not walk. If I couldn't walk I would not be able to work. Now I can walk pain-free again. You are my savior! I am so grateful. Thank you!"

CHEST PAIN AND FIBROID TUMORS

"All my life I have been in pain. Now, I feel wonderful."

Kaitlin is a nurse. She had experienced severe and unrelenting pain in her upper chest all her life. There was no known medical cause found, even after every type of medical test had been conducted. She also had dreadful pain in her lower abdomen due to two inoperable fibroid tumors. After her first healing session, the pain in her upper chest left completely. After the second, the intolerable pain in her lower abdomen disappeared.

Kaitlin says, "Now I feel wonderful! Thank you!"

There are, of course, many, many more anecdotes covering almost every imaginable type of malady, but this is all the room we have for now. As the authority on energy healing, I hope that you have found this chapter to be helpful as an introduction to such an expansive metaphysical topic. The concepts may be new to you, although the principles have always been used, in every part of the world, throughout history.

If you feel that I may be able to assist you or a loved one, please call me in Toronto at 416-447-9550. If there is a good fit with us and we do work together, I will visit you in the privacy of your own home and I will commit to working with you until you are completely well again. In the meantime, may blessings of Love and Light always be upon you.

Thank you for your interest! You can learn more at www.PhilipYoungHealer.com

Save My Relationship

The Master Plan for Creating an Amazing Relationship

CHRIS HART

Beata came to me with her relationship in tatters. Her boyfriend, Matt, had recently moved out of the flat they'd shared for five years, claiming that he no longer loved her. She thought they had been moving towards marriage and was utterly devastated, lost, and confused. She told me that I was her last option. I hear that a lot. Beata did not believe that she could rekindle the relationship with Matt. She thought it was a lost cause and that she was a lost cause, too. She was grasping at straws. I saw a woman whose self-esteem and confidence were at an all-time low. I saw a woman who was broken, emotionally. I saw a woman I could help.

I welcomed Beata with open arms. We sat down and, as I listened to her talk, I formulated an action plan for her to follow. She stuck with the plan, and with me, through many months of emotional healing and relationship work. I am thrilled to say that Beata and Matt are now happily married! Beata succeeded because she realized that she needed to work on healing herself as well as her relationship. Do not think this was an easy task for Beata. Some of the things I had to say were not easy for her to hear. My job is to be real. I will not tell you what you want to hear; I am not here to stroke your ego. Healing does not occur within denial. Beata had to do some difficult self-healing before we tackled her relational-healing with Matt. She is now extremely confident and aligned with her feelings. Furthermore, she is happily married and pursuing a life of "happily ever after."

If you are struggling with a failed, or near-failing, relationship, I can help you, too. My methods are not traditional self-help methodology, which focus on the mind. My methods focus on the heart; I concentrate on emotional guidance. You did not enter into your relationship using your mind. On the day you met your mate you did not think to yourself, "He seems like a good fit. I think I'll develop a loving relationship with this one." No, you did not use your mind; you used your heart. You met and fell in love. Therefore, you cannot solve relational problems with your head. This is an emotional problem that requires heart healing.

Maybe you wish to rekindle a romance that is dwindling, but you aren't quite ready for marriage. Such was the case with Talia, who came to me during a troubling time in her life. She was young and in love...or so she thought. Her boyfriend, Doug, had recently distanced himself from her. At first, he pulled away emotionally. He still hung out with her and took her out, but he seemed distracted and was not fully present with her. Eventually, he began making plans that did not include Talia. She was left feeling hurt and confused. Talia's thoughts began to take over her conscious moments with a constant barrage of questions: Was Doug the right choice for her? Should she wait for him to come around and decide what he wants and who he wants to be with? Should she move on and date someone else? Exactly what was he doing when he was not with her?

Talia's friends were divided. Some counseled her to not let Doug get away; they gave her ideas of how she could change herself to be more attractive to Doug. Others scoffed at that notion and told Talia she could do better than Doug, and counted off several other guys who'd already expressed interest in dating Talia. Talia's mother told her that "Things have a way of working themselves out" and to be patient. Talia's head was spinning from overthinking this situation.

Talia eventually got out of her own head and contacted me. After our first session, Talia was able to organize her thoughts and set them aside to focus on her heart. Soon she realized that she was not quite ready to give up on Doug. She was not sure if the relationship was one that would last forever, but she wanted to pursue it. So, we set to work.

I soon realized that Talia was harboring quite a bit of anger, not only towards Doug, but towards the friends who had been so quick to tell her what to do. Of course, this really means that Talia was angry with herself for allowing others to treat her this way. She denied this in the beginning; I had to be quite stern with her to enable her to see how she was allowing others to treat her. Talia was young, a college student, so her friends held a lot of influence over her. So often I find that people care more about what others think of them than what they think of themselves! Eventually, Talia came to see that she had to stop listening to others and only listen to me, and herself.

We put an action plan in place and Talia was able to examine her heart, rather than being lost in her thoughts all the time. After working with me, Talia was able to emotionally heal herself. She is now a much stronger young woman who has many close friends, yet thinks for herself. Thanks to my work, Doug has decided that he wants to continue his relationship with Talia. He is much more open with her about what he is wants. Talia and Doug are now happily dating and are excited to see where their relationship goes in the future.

When you utilize my methods you will find the last missing jigsaw piece that solves everything in your world of romance; that is, your relationship. I will enable you to regain your confidence and self-esteem by giving you the knowledge of what you can do to resolve your romantic problems. Many women come to me for help. My methods work because I am a man, therefore I think like a man. I can help women understand how their men think.

One of the first things a woman does when her relationship hits the rocks is to pick up the phone and call her closest friend or family member. After all, your friends will commiserate with you and offer you a shoulder to cry on. On the other hand, be cautious because your loved ones may soon begin to belittle your man or point out everything that was wrong with the relationship. This is no good! Whether they are correct or not, they are not in your shoes. They are not living your life, nor do they understand what you feel or what you want. You should stop listening to friends and family, especially if what they are saying does not align with your desires. They usually mean well, but cannot understand your relationship or your heart.

Once you stop listening to others, you must next stop overthinking. Putting an end to overthinking is the key! If you are hurting and mourning the loss of your love, you are thinking, thinking, thinking about what you can do to get him back, or what you wish you had done differently. You are spending too much time and energy thinking about your problems. All of this overthinking is surely affecting other areas of your life. Are you able to be productive at work? Or do make careless mistakes along the way because you are focused on your current loss. Are you fully present when someone else is talking to you? Or is your mind on your own problems that you are feverishly thinking about? Are you losing sleep due to overthinking? Overthinking about your current romantic problems leads to self-blame, loss of confidence, and a lack of awareness of the true nature of the problem. Two people usually share the blame when a relationship ends. When you overthink, you victimize yourself. Do not think like a victim. I will teach you how to become a victor. With my new way of thinking, you will be put back in control of your emotions.

Having control over your emotions is the key to victory. I will teach you how to have closure with the old self and to be the woman in control. Controlling your emotions can change you completely. You may not recognize this change in yourself, but others will see this metamorphosis and be inspired by you. People will be attracted to you because of your inner transformation. Learning to become the victor and think like a victor requires that you get real with yourself. You must look deeply into your own desires and motives to recognize things that need to be changed. Consider me your personal coach; I will "kick butt" if I sense that you are being too soft on yourself, just as any good coach does with his or her trainee. I want you to succeed, therefore I will not accept anything less than 100% from you. If you are just looking for someone who will stroke your ego and tell you that you are always right, you may wish to go back to your friends. I am not that person. I am the person who will affect real change in your life and in your relationships.

There is beautiful change to be had, if you are willing to make it. If my relationship were ending, I would be wondering what I could have done to change things or save the relationship. Regrets would always be there somewhere. Women with regrets cry. Do you have regrets? Successful women do not cry; they try. In fact, they make things happen. Women who take action have no regrets. You, too, can make things happen to solve your relationship problems.

When a woman comes to my practice, the first thing I ask her is this: Do you really want him back? This may sound like an empty question, but it is not. The answer to this question is incredibly important. Often, women do not know the true answer to this question when they first come to see me. If you only want him back in order to exact revenge on him for the way he treated you, my methods will not work. You must be sure that you want him back and that you want him back for the right reasons. The second question I ask is this: To what degree do you want this man back in your life?

Sometimes a woman comes to me and does not know the answer to those questions. I met with Carla and could tell right away that she was unsure about seeing me. She was unsure about many things. Once we cleared the air with incense and began to set aside her thoughts and focus on her heart, Carla realized that she held too much anger and resentment towards her boyfriend to continue a relationship with him. She had been blinding herself to this reality because she was afraid of what to do without him.

Carla was so afraid of being on her own that she was willing to chase after a failing relationship. She was so caught up in her thoughts that she did not even realize what this was doing to her heart. Carla was putting herself last and discounting her own feelings!

I quickly formulated an action plan for Carla. She chose not to pursue the failing relationship with her boyfriend; rather, she chose to pursue the failing relationship with herself. I got real with her and coached her on how to put herself first in her heart. This does not mean that she was to become a narcissist! No, this meant that she had to re-learn how to love and care for herself. She also had to learn to let go of her boyfriend. Using my methods, Carla was able to heal herself emotionally.

Carla recently contacted me to let me know that she is dating someone new. She is in love! She breathlessly told me how her new beau was the perfect match for her. I smiled to myself because I know he is the perfect match for her because she healed herself and was open to finding love.

Maybe you will decide that you do not want your man back in your life. Maybe you will decide that you want your man back for the right reasons and you realize to what degree you want him in your life. I can help you with both situations. When you work with me, I ask that you listen only to two people: yourself and me. Please do not think I am being conceited with this statement. If you are having a problem with a guy, listen to me. I do not say this to sound conceited, but I am a guy. Since I am a guy, I think like a guy. You need someone who thinks like a guy to help you with your guy. Furthermore, I have your best interest in mind. I have no preconceived notions about your relationship or whether the man is 'good enough' for you. I want what you want.

Listen to yourself. Have you been doing that? Or have you been overthinking the problem and assigning all kinds of blame to yourself? Listen to your authentic self. Do not allow others to influence your thoughts. It matters what you think and what you want, not what the others in your life think or want. Once you are ready to stop overthinking and blaming, you are ready for productive change.

I will share a bit of what I can do with you to save your relationship. First, I use incense to clear any negativity in the air. I know which incense to use that will combine the right energy with the right purpose of healing your relationship. Incense also prepares your mind for the process of healing your relationship. The incense I use will heighten your awareness, focus your thoughts, and bring about calm or healing energies during our work. When using incense to enhance energy, it provides assistance to direct your energy in a specific direction of self-healing. You will ultimately be able to alter your inner perceptions about yourself to create the life you want. Of course incense cannot do this alone, but it can help create or enhance the desired energies for our work together.

Along with incense, I use crystals in my practice. Crystals have the power to heal and attract if used wisely. Rose Quartz is a particularly good crystal for healing relationships, and is one that I use in my practice. Rose Quartz, also known as the Love Stone, is the stone of unconditional love; therefore, it is particularly powerful for healing broken relationships. Rose Quartz opens the heart chakra to encourage forgiveness and will, along with my counseling, help you let go of anger, resentment, jealousy, or any negative feelings you have towards your partner.

We begin with the first of two tests. These 'tests' will determine my unique action plan for your situation. The first test involves the use of imagery. Imagine your guy standing right in front of you. Take time to allow his image to materialize in your mind, noting details of his appearance. After you have the image of him in mind, ask yourself what colour you feel he has near his head area. Next, ask yourself what colour he has in his heart area. Finally, ask yourself what colour he has in his erogenous area. Take your time and allow the colours to materialize. Now take a look at yourself. What colours do you see in these areas for yourself? If you are struggling with this imagery while reading, do not lose heart. When you visit with me, I will guide you to accurately see the colours you have in mind for yourself and your partner.

Colour is, at its most essential, light and energy. People have been using colour, along with light and energy, to heal for thousands of years. Colour is also a form of nonverbal communication that influences emotion. There is a specific psychological response to each colour. Psychological effects have been observed relating to the following two main categories of colour: warm and cool. Warm colours, such as red, yellow, and orange, can spark a variety of emotions ranging from comfort and warmth to hostility and anger. Cool colours, such as green, blue and purple, often spark feelings of calmness and peace, as well as sadness or melancholy.

The colours you saw in the above exercise indicate your emotions regarding yourself and your mate. Your colour choices guide me in developing your personal action plan to harmonize the colours into the proper colour for a successful, loving relationship. If your colour choices indicate that your relationship is in real danger of ending, I can work with you to change the colours you see.

I will teach you to use your mind and emotions to align your proper colour with your guy. Along with incense and crystals, I utilize a picture of the person, since a photograph is an inner vibration of a person. Once you start working on your colours with me, relational changes occur quickly. A woman I counseled recently was able to complete an emotional bonding with her guy, even though he had moved out and ended the relationship. This couple is now married.

I hope that I have inspired you to take action to salvage a hurting relationship. If you are ready to take charge of your life and save your relationship, contact me through my website: www.loveguidance.co.uk. My hope is that reading this has been an awakening for you to see your own problems as they truly are, and to stop thinking like a victim. Through a session with me, you will be able to regain your strength and confidence to win him over. I will help you find closure with your old self and what has gone wrong in your past. Your new way of thinking will attract people to you and put you back in control of yourself and your emotions.

Do not be a woman with regret; be a woman in control.

Bringing Balance
to Your Life

DENNIS GARRIDO

When I woke up in the hospital staring up into the terrified eyes of someone I cared about, after my second cardiac arrest in one year, I knew that things had to change in my life. Especially because I was only in my twenties at the time.

Everything in my life was out of balance. Obviously, physically because I was lying in the emergency room, but more importantly my mind, emotions, and spirit were completely out of whack, and that had taken a toll on my body.

Now you may be wondering how someone so young could have had two cardiac arrests before the age of 30? It won't be hard to imagine once I share my story with you. I wish I could tell you that I had a great upbringing, one filled with laughter and love, but it wasn't.

At age eleven I was removed from my parent's home by The Children's Aid Society because they deemed my parents unfit to raise me. During that time, I went through a whirlwind of emotions. A part of me was happy that change was finally occurring, because clearly at that point, the way things were, wasn't working at all.

Another part of me felt fear because of the unknown. I didn't know exactly where I would be living, nor did I know for sure what my group & foster homes would be like, what the other kids would be like, what the living conditions would be like, how far or close I'd be to my family and hometown, etc. Essentially, I wasn't 100% certain nor 100% convinced that I was going into better circumstances.

Also, I felt sad, since I wouldn't see my parents or siblings anymore, nor my home town and many of the people whom I'd see on a regular basis; everything FAMILIAR would be gone! Lastly, I felt angry, that it had come to me being removed from my parent's house, away from those who were in my life for all those years. As twisted and messed up as it may be, I was angry that I was leaving a life that I had become accustomed to and felt somewhat comfortable in (comfortable in comparison to the unknown that lay ahead); and most of all, angry that I was leaving FAMILIARITY!!!!

Please understand me, I am no longer angry at my parents, and you shouldn't be either. They did the best they could, but when you are broken yourself, unless you find a way out, you will repeat what had been bestowed on you from the previous generations. I can be thankful because what I went through helped create the person I am today and as a coach, it gives me great empathy and understanding to be able to help others. So, don't feel sorry for me because even though my life had a rough start, I get to choose the rest of it and it is going to be GREAT!!!

THE NEXT SEVEN YEARS OF MY LIFE

For the next seven years until I turned 18, I was bounced from foster/group home to foster/group home. I rarely spent more than three months at any one place, and it caused some major emotional setbacks that took me a long time to overcome.

One of the biggest negative emotional setbacks was again to do with familiarity. As I spent time with those at my new home, seeing them every day and coming to know them personally; I naturally formed a connection/friendship with them. It seemed that no sooner had I done that; they were removed from my life. People whom I really liked (a few of them, whom I loved), ALL GONE!!! Which basically solidified my already ingrained defence mechanism of keeping distant from others; not allowing anyone to get close enough to form any connection with me.

Inevitably, this made it very difficult for me to form any type of relationship with anyone. School and extracurricular activities were hard because I never knew how long I would be staying in one place. What was the point of making friends if I could never keep them? It was a lot easier to keep my distance than to reach out yet again and have everything torn away from me.

Eventually, I started to tear down the wall that prevented me from getting too close to anyone. To this day, the negative emotional setbacks I experienced, still affect me to some degree; though I CHOOSE not to allow them to prevent me from forming meaningful relationships!

THE DARKEST TIME OF MY LIFE

All that change led to one of the darkest periods of my life. Emotionally and mentally I had shut down and could no longer function. Life was so hard. Even things that were simple, now became agonizingly difficult and it hit the point where I didn't want to live anymore. What was the use of carrying on in this horrible life when there wasn't any hope of it changing?

My life began to narrow down to one permanent solution, and that was to end it all by committing suicide. I just couldn't handle life anymore, but I truly believe that Almighty God, the universe or whatever you want to call it, had a bigger plan for me. Even though I tried several times, I just couldn't die!!! Because of those attempts, I ended up in psychiatric institutions, a few times.

It finally came to the point where I was tired of trying to die, I was tired of institutions and I was weary from all the self-harm, and so I came to a decision. I guess you could say that it was a turning point in my life; I wasn't going to attempt suicide anymore. I wasn't sure what to do because my circumstances hadn't changed, but I was willing to look for options. That was the beginning point of change in my life. The will to live!!!

IT DIDN'T GET BETTER RIGHT AWAY

Life is a journey with twists, hills, and valleys of varying shapes and sizes, with occasional points where you make decisions that put you on a different path. The determination not to kill myself had set me on a new road, but I still didn't know what to do or which way to go. It was slow going as I fumbled my way through, but at least I was moving forward!!!

At age 18 I was no longer in the custody of The Children's Aid Society, so, I moved back with my parents, which was the perfect testing grounds for me to apply the life lessons I had learned so far. You would be amazed by how much maturity one can have at 18 when you have been through what I have. It wasn't easy, and it was hard work, but I managed to re-establish a relationship with my parents and not only complete high school, but also graduate from post-secondary schooling.

One of the things I had decided to do was get my student loans paid off in the six-month grace period, which I managed to do; but in doing so, I pushed myself way beyond my physical limits which brought on the first cardiac arrest.

You would think I would have learned from that first experience, but I didn't, and less than a year later we are back to the beginning of this chapter waking up in the hospital from my second one.

This time I learned my lesson and chose a different path, but I still didn't know how to achieve what I needed. For so long I had lived in imbalance, that I didn't know where to start, but the catalyst for change was just around the corner.

I FINALLY REALIZED WHAT BALANCE WAS

Believe it or not, it is the simplest things that can bring about the most profound changes in life. My search for balance in my life had begun, and it is amazing how the answer came; by a knock at my door one day.

That day I was busy working on something, so when the first knock came, I ignored it. It was only after a couple of rings of the doorbell that I finally decided that I would answer it. There was a well-dressed gentleman at the door and even though I don't remember most of what he said, one thing became clear, I was missing an essential element to finding the balance I craved. Now, I knew what it was. You can only find balance when you address ALL the areas of your life, and I had been missing one. The spiritual side.

It is amazing what happens when you finally have all the pieces together. As I started to study the Bible, I finally could build a solid spiritual foundation, that enabled me to re-evaluate things in my life, and thus, put a plan together to create balance in my life. In the rest of this chapter, I am going to share with you what I learned.

Just before I do that, I do want to mention one thing. All of this is a process. Can I say that I am 100% balanced in my life? No, but when I started at **3-4%** and then jumped to 85%, I think that is very good growth. It's difficult to attain 100% balance in every aspect of one's life, that is why even the most successful people keep learning and growing. So, the goal is not perfection, but growth. As long as you are continuing to move forward, that is all that matters.

7 STEPS TO BRING BALANCE TO YOUR LIFE

Here's one of the things that I have learned about bringing balance to your life. In some ways, it is easy. The steps I am going to teach you are simple to understand. The hard part is training yourself to be aware of it every day and live by it. The good thing is, though it may be hard at first, the more you practice it, the easier it gets.

STEP 1

Ask yourself, "What are my priorities in life?" You want to look at it from all aspects of your life, personal and professional. In terms of personal that includes goals physically, emotionally, mentally, spiritually, relationships (such as your spouse or significant other), family and friends. You want to look at it from the point of what you need and what you want. For each one, you should have one to two priorities.

In terms of professional, they can include your current work situation and areas of improvement there, plus plan for your future. Put down both needs and wants.

	NEEDS	WANTS
P E R S O N A L		
P R O F E S S I O N A L		

STEP 2

Look at your needs column. What are the most important priorities personally and professionally? It is important that you only start out working on a few at a time. If you try to do everything at once, you will become overwhelmed and quit. Then, figure out the things you need to do to get those needs met.

STEP 3

Now go through your wants and do the same thing as Step 2 above. Don't overlook this. Part of having balance in life is having both your needs and wants met. Obviously, your needs are more important, but without the wants, you give up hope.

STEP 4

Set up a timeline for those needs to be accomplished. What are you going to do today, this week, this month, this year, and in the next five years to bring yourself to reach those priorities?

STEP 5

Do the same thing for your wants. Set up your timeline of completion.

STEP 6

DO THE ACTIONS. Here is where the rubber meets the road. You can plan and plan and plan, but if there is no action involved you will be in the same place, with the same problems, five years from now.

STEP 7

Re-evaluate. Every few months go back through this whole process again.

As you grow and change, so will your priorities, your needs and your wants.

THE BEST WAY TO ACCOMPLISH THIS

Very rarely can a person accomplish this alone. Have you ever heard the saying, "You can't see the forest for the trees?" That is what happens in our lives. We get so caught up in the unimportant things right in front of us, that we miss the big picture and we don't recognize growth when it occurs.

Now, you do have several options. One is to have family members try to help you through this. While you do need their support, they are usually looking at the same trees you are and can miss things.

Two, you can go to friends for help. They do tend to see more of the big picture, but many times they can't give you the encouragement and motivation you need at times to get past yourself.

Three, you work with a professional who knows how to help you bring balance to your life. They can come alongside of you and guide you to the quickest path to success because there will be obstacles that try to stop you. Did I forget to mention that?

No road to balance is smooth; little pebbles will get into your shoes to irritate you and take your focus off your goals. Barriers will be put up that you will have to learn how to go over, under, around or through. People will get in your way and tell you that it is the wrong road to take and you should follow them. All sorts of things will try to keep you from what you want.

Coaches are keen observers who can not only help you with what is going on right now, but they have been down your road and they know what is up ahead and can keep you moving forward, even when everything is telling you to stop.

That is what I'm offering to be for you. Let me help you on your path to balance in your life. I have been on both sides of the coin, and I can guide you through the roughest parts. I can relate to what you are feeling and am more than willing to help you navigate this wonderful thing called life.

First of all, if you would like more information on how to start this process, you can pre-order my upcoming book at www.dennisgarrido.com Second, you can email me at dennis@dennisgarrido.com and request your free 15-minute phone consultation where we can discuss your situation and see if we are a good fit for each other. Third, maybe you realize more people need to hear this message. I am also available to speak to groups and conferences. If so, just send me an email, and we can arrange a time to speak.

No matter what you decide, know this. You can achieve balance in your life. It is possible. I can tell you that it has been worth everything I went through to get to this point. The peace I experience now, compared to the chaos I lived before, is so amazing and I wish the same for you.

Don't miss out. Make the choice to change your life today, and I guarantee that you won't regret it!!!